DENTAL ASSISTING
COLORING BOOK

Donna J. Phinney, CDA, BA, M. Ed.
Spokane Community College

Judy H. Halstead, CDA, BA
Spokane Community College

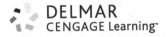

DELMAR
CENGAGE Learning™

Australia • Brazil • Japan • Korea • Mexico • Singapore • Spain • United Kingdom • United States

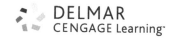

Dental Assisting Coloring Book
Donna J. Phinney and Judy H. Halstead

Vice President, Career and Professional Editorial: Dave Garza

Director of Learning Solutions: Matthew Kane

Acquisitions Editor: Tari Broderick

Managing Editor: Marah Bellegarde

Senior Product Manager: Darcy M. Scelsi

Editorial Assistant: Ian Lewis

Vice President, Career and Professional Marketing: Jennifer McAvey

Marketing Manager: Kristin McNary

Marketing Coordinator: Erica Ropitsky

Production Director: Carolyn Miller

Production Manager: Andrew Crouth

Content Project Management: PreMediaGlobal

Senior Art Director: Jack Pendleton

For product information and technology assistance, contact us at
Cengage Learning Customer & Sales Support, 1-800-354-9706

For permission to use material from this text or product,
submit all requests online at **www.cengage.com/permissions.**
Further permissions questions can be e-mailed to
permissionrequest@cengage.com

Library of Congress Control Number: 2010925127

ISBN-13: 978-1-4390-5931-9

ISBN-10: 1-4390-5931-4

Delmar
5 Maxwell Drive
Clifton Park, NY 12065-2919
USA

Cengage Learning is a leading provider of customized learning solutions with office locations around the globe, including Singapore, the United Kingdom, Australia, Mexico, Brazil, and Japan. Locate your local office at: **www.cengage.com/global**

Cengage Learning products are represented in Canada by Nelson Education, Ltd.

To learn more about Delmar, visit **www.cengage.com/delmar**

Purchase any of our products at your local college store or at our preferred online store **www.cengagebrain.com**

Notice to the Reader

Publisher does not warrant or guarantee any of the products described herein or perform any independent analysis in connection with any of the product information contained herein. Publisher does not assume, and expressly disclaims, any obligation to obtain and include information other than that provided to it by the manufacturer. The reader is expressly warned to consider and adopt all safety precautions that might be indicated by the activities described herein and to avoid all potential hazards. By following the instructions contained herein, the reader willingly assumes all risks in connection with such instructions. The publisher makes no representations or warranties of any kind, including but not limited to, the warranties of fitness for particular purpose or merchantability, nor are any such representations implied with respect to the material set forth herein, and the publisher takes no responsibility with respect to such material. The publisher shall not be liable for any special, consequential, or exemplary damages resulting, in whole or part, from the readers' use of, or reliance upon, this material.

Printed at CLDPC, USA, 04-24

Table of Contents

General Anatomy

Basic Cell Structures

Label and color the structures on the illustration.

Match the structure to the definition.

1. _____ nucleus   A. the outer wall of the cell

2. _____ chromosomes   B. makes up all of the substance of the cell minus
                                   the nucleus

3. _____ cell membrane   C. controlling body of the cell

4. _____ cytoplasm   D. contain DNA and transmit genetic information

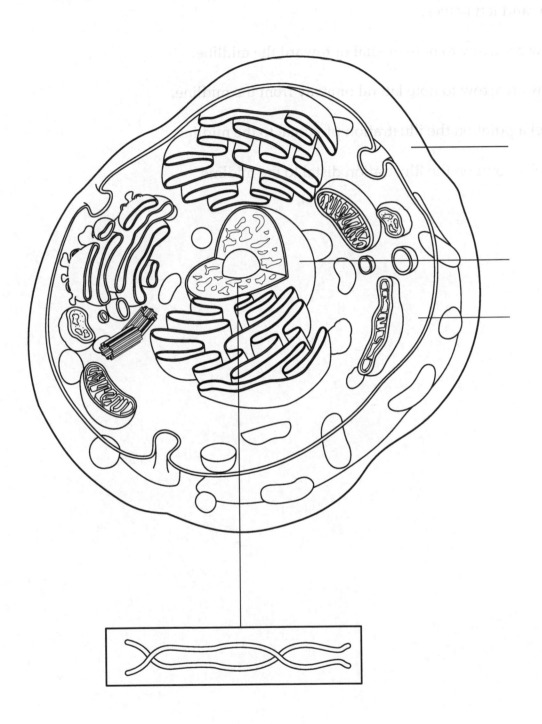

Body Planes

Draw the sagittal plane in black. Recall that the sagittal plane divides the body into right and left halves.

Draw an arrow to note medial or toward the midline.

Draw an arrow to note lateral or away from the midline.

Label a point on the illustration proximal to the midline.

Label a point on the illustration distal to the midline.

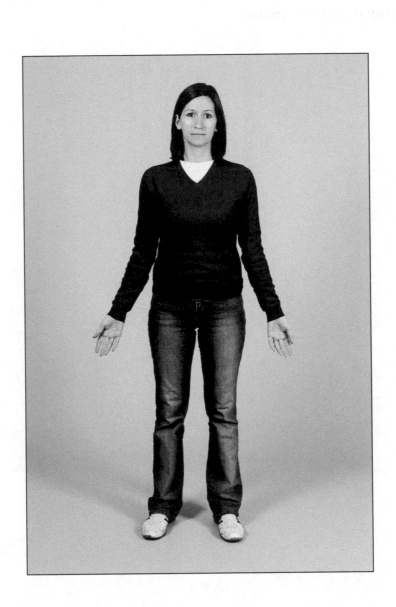

Body Directions

Draw a red line indicating the frontal plane. Draw arrows indicating anterior and posterior to the frontal plane.

Draw a black line indicating the tranverse plane. Draw arrows indicating superior and inferior to the transverse plane.

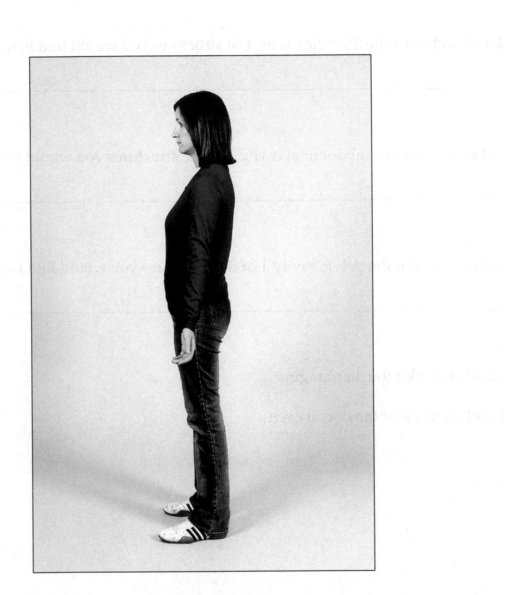

Body Cavities

List the two sections the body cavities are divided into.

_____

Label and color the thoracic cavity. List structures you would find here.

_____

Label and color the abdominal cavity. List the structures you would find here.

_____

Label and color the pelvic cavity. List the structures you would find here.

_____

Label and color the diaphragm.

Label the parts of the dorsal cavity.

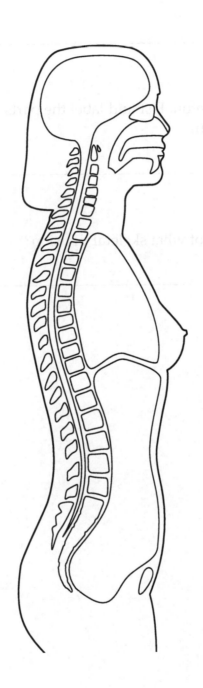

Axial and Appendicular Skeleton

Color the axial skeleton. List and label the parts of the skeleton that make up the axial division.

_____

Color the appendicular skeleton. List and label the parts of the skeleton that make up the appendicular division.

_____

The hands and feet are part of what skeletal division?

_____

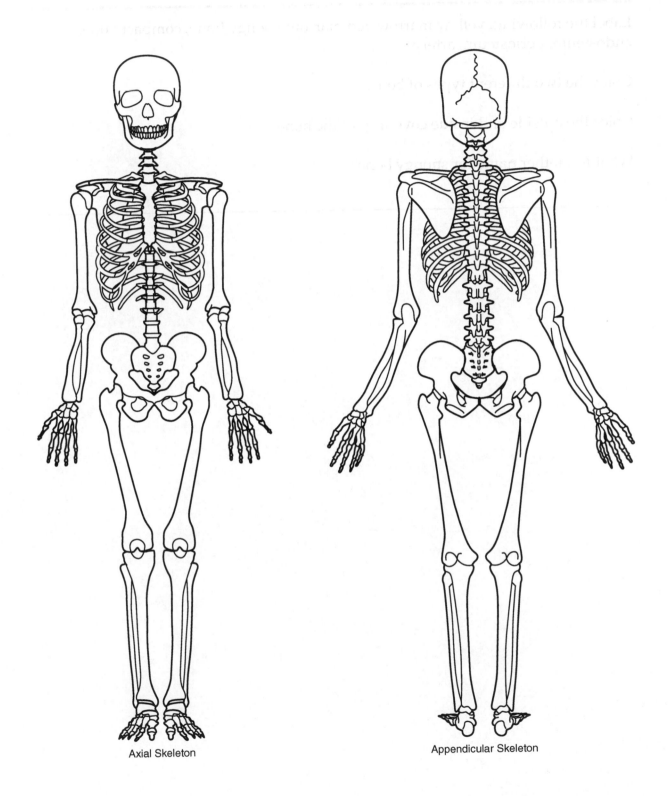

Axial Skeleton

Appendicular Skeleton

Anatomic Features of the Bone

Label the following: yellow marrow, red marrow, spongy bone, compact bone, endosteum, periosteum, artery.

Color the two different types of bone.

Color the outside and inside coverings of the bone.

What is another name for spongy bone?

_____

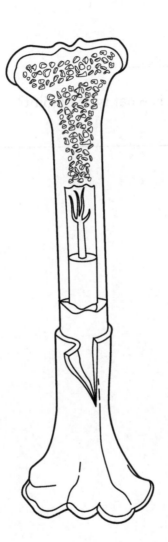

Skeletal Joints

Label and color the ball and socket joint.

Label and color the hinge joint.

Label and color the temporomandibular joint.

Identify the synovial joint.

Another name for "joints" is _____.

The temporomandibular joint is what type of joint?

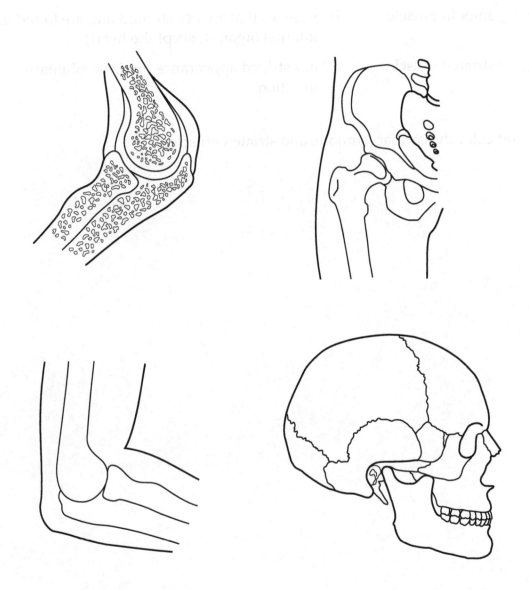

Types of Muscle Tissue

Match the type of muscle tissue to the definition.

1. _____ cardiac muscle

2. _____ smooth muscle

3. _____ striated muscle

A. long thin muscles that have stripes and are sometimes called "skeletal" muscles

B. muscles that are not striated and are found in internal organs (except the heart)

C. has striped appearance but is involuntary in action

Label and color the cardiac, smooth, and striated muscles.

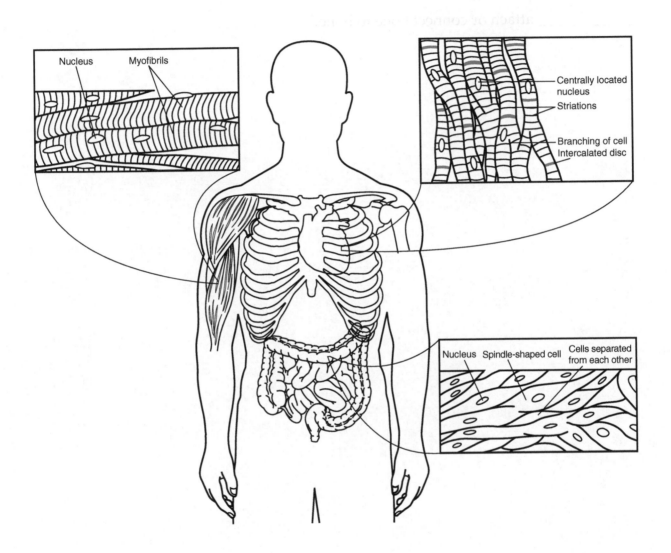

Tendons and Ligaments

Label and color the tendons.

Label and color the ligament.

_____ attach muscle to bone.

_____ attach or connect bone to bone.

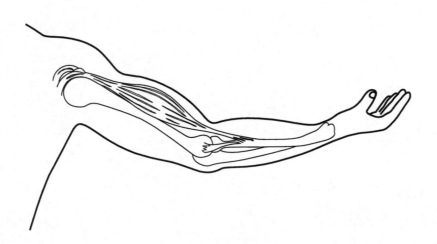

Structure of a Neuron

Label and color the following: axon, beads of myelin, dendrites, nucleus, neuron cell body.

Draw an arrow on the nerve fibers that conduct impulses away from the nerve cell.

Draw an arrow on the nerve fibers that conduct impulses toward the nerve cell.

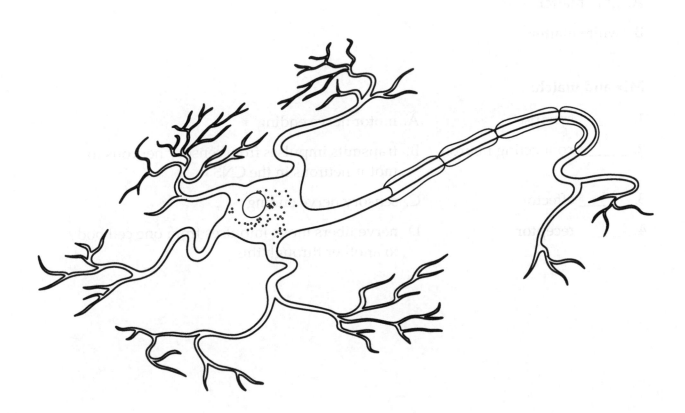

Simple Reflex Arc

Draw an arrow tracing the path of impulse through the spinal cord and back for a response.

Label and color the following: axon, cell body, connecting (associative) neuron, gray matter, motor nerve ending, motor neuron, sensory nerve ending, sensory neuron, spinal cord, and synapse.

Where are the connecting neurons located? _____

A. gray matter

B. white matter

Mix and match:

1. _____ synapse

2. _____ connecting neuron

3. _____ effector

4. _____ receptor

A. motor nerve ending

B. transmits impulses from sensory neurons to motor neurons in the CNS

C. sensory nerve ending

D. nerve fibers move impulses from one cell body to another through this

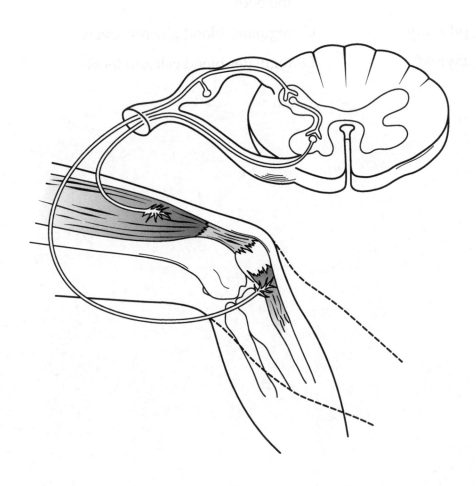

Structures of the Endocrine System

Locate, label, and color all structures of the endocrine system.

Match the structure to the function.

1. _____ adrenal

A. controls the actions of most other glands

2. _____ pancreas

B. regulates stress hormones and water content of the body

3. _____ pituitary

C. regulates blood glucose levels

4. _____ thyroid

D. regulates blood calcium levels

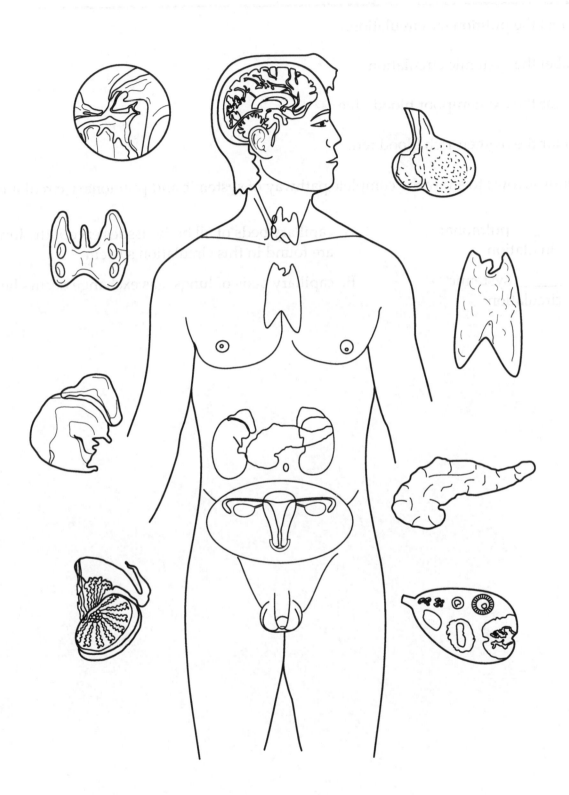

System and Pulmonary Circulation

Label the pulmonary circulation.

Label the systemic circulation.

Color the oxygen-poor blood blue.

Color the oxygen-rich blood red.

Draw arrows to show the complete pathway of systemic and pulmonary circulation.

1. _____ pulmonary circulation

2. _____ systemic circulation

A. capillary beds of all body tissues except the lungs are found in this circulation system

B. capillary beds of lungs, gas exchange occurs here

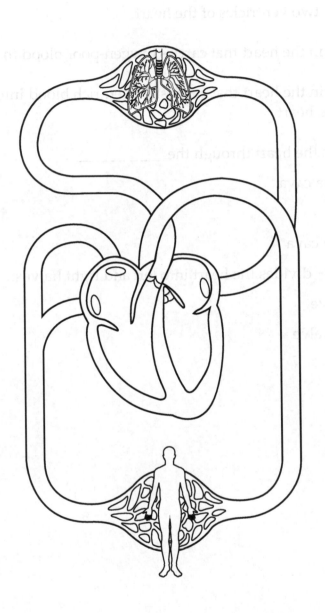

Structures of the Heart

Label and color the four valves of the heart.

Label and color the two atriums of the heart.

Label and color the two ventricles of the heart.

Color the pathway in the heart that carries oxygen-poor blood to the lungs.

Color the pathway in the heart that carries oxygen-rich blood into the heart from the lungs and out of the heart.

1. The blood leaves the heart through the _____.

   A. superior vena cava

   B. aorta

   C. inferior vena cava

2. The _____ divides the heart into left and right halves.

   A. bicuspid valve

   B. pulmonary valve

   C. septum

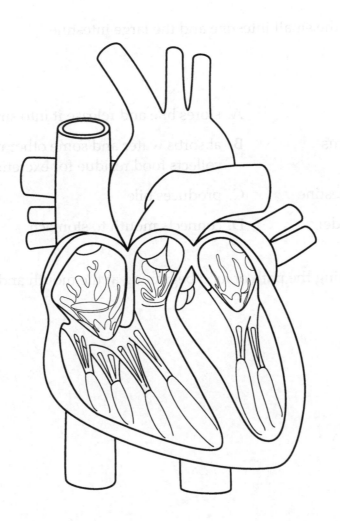

Structures of the Digestive System

List and identify the following: large intestine, small intestine, pancreas, liver, mouth, stomach, esophagus, gallbladder, and salivary glands.

Outline and color the liver, gall bladder, pancreas, and stomach.

Outline and color the mouth, esophagus, and salivary glands.

Outline and color the small intestine and the large intestine.

Mix and match:

1. _____ liver

2. _____ esophagus

3. _____ large intestine

4. _____ gallbladder

A. stores bile and release it into small intestine

B. absorbs water and some other nutrients, and collects food residue for excretion

C. produces bile

D. connects mouth to stomach

Draw a line following the path of food beginning at the mouth and ending at the large intestine.

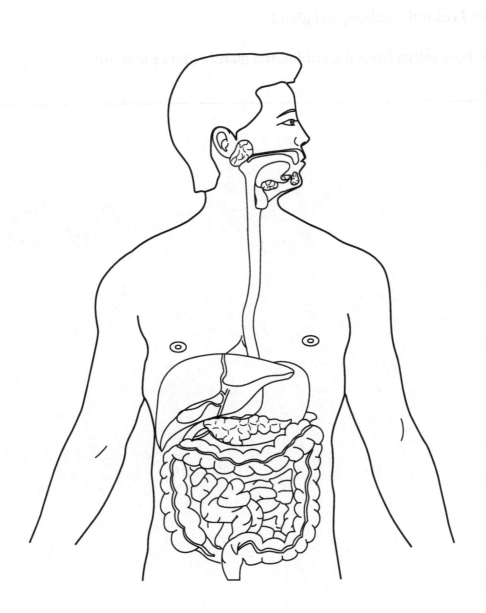

Salivary Glands and Ducts

Locate and color the parotid gland and Stensen's duct.

Locate and color the submandibular gland and Wharton's duct.

Locate and color the sublingual gland.

Describe how saliva from the sublingual gland enters the mouth.

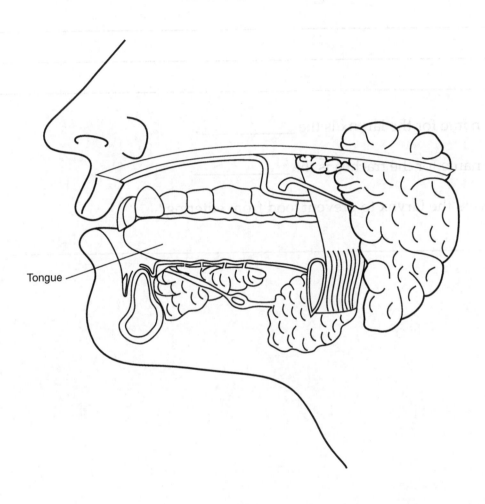

Tongue

Structures of the Respiratory System

Label and color the sinuses and nasal cavity.

Label and color the epiglottis, pharynx, larynx, and trachea.

Label and color the pulmonary vein and pulmonary artery.

List the structures that make up the bronchial tree.

_____

_____

_____

Another name for the larynx is the _____.

Another name for the trachea is the _____.

What covers the larynx to prevent food from entering?

_____

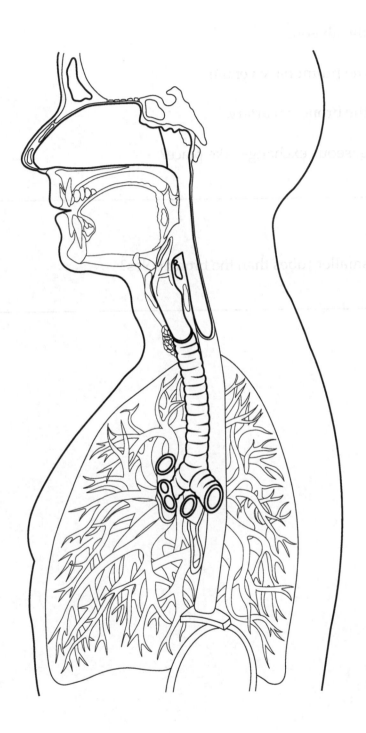

Structures of the Bronchi

Label and color the bronchiole.

Label and color the alveoli.

Label and color the pulmonary venule.

Label and color the bronchial artery.

Where does the gaseous exchange take place?

_____

Are the bronchi smaller tubes than the bronchioles?

_____

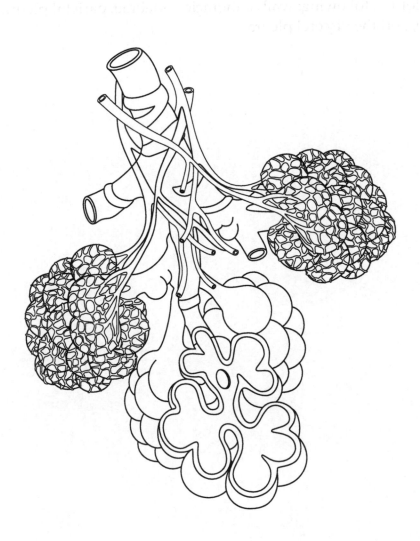

The Lungs

The lungs lie between what two structures when looking at this cross-section?

_____

Label and color the following: wall of thoracic vertebrae, parietal pleura, pleural space, and the visceral pleura.

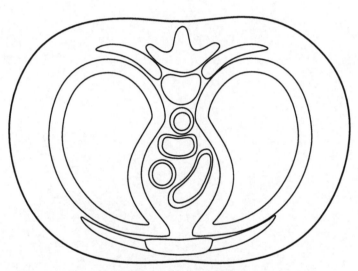

Horizontal cross section of the lungs

Tonsils

Label and color the uvula.

Label and color the hard palate and the soft palate.

Label and color the palatine tonsils, lingual tonsils, and pharyngeal tonsils.

Mix and match:

1. _____ lingual tonsils   A. on the posterior wall of the nasopharynx

2. _____ palatine tonsils   B. on the base of the tongue

3. _____ pharyngeal tonsils   C. on each side of the throat

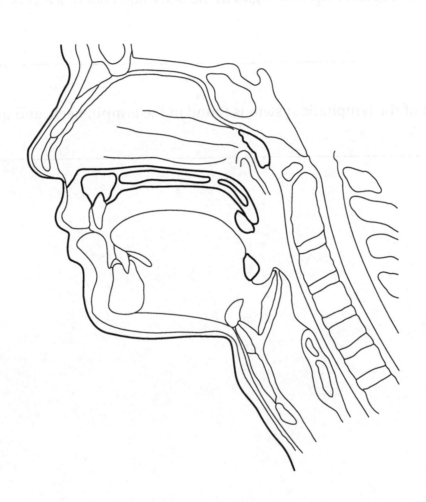

The Immune System

Label and color the organs from the lymphatic system.

Label and color the tissue from the skeletal system.

Label and color the digestive system.

1. Which is the largest lymphoid organ in the body and contains a very rich blood supply?

   _____

2. What part of the lymphatic system is found in the armpit, neck, and groin areas?

   _____

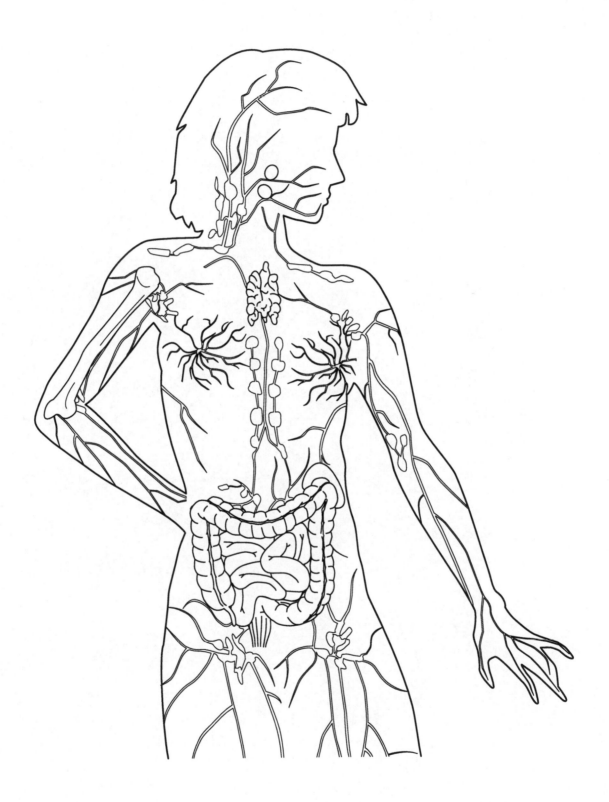

Head and Neck Anatomy

Landmarks of the Face

Identify the landmarks on the picture, draw a circle around each landmark, and then color in each area. Landmarks include: ala of the nose, labial commissure, labiomental groove, labial tubercle, nasolabial groove, philtrum, vermilion border, and vermilion zone.

Match the structure to the definition.

1. _____ nasolabial groove

2. _____ philtrum

3. _____ labial commissure

4. _____ vermilion zone

A. corners of the mouth

B. shallow V-shaped depression above the upper lip

C. reddish portion of the lips

D. ala of the nose to the corners of the mouth

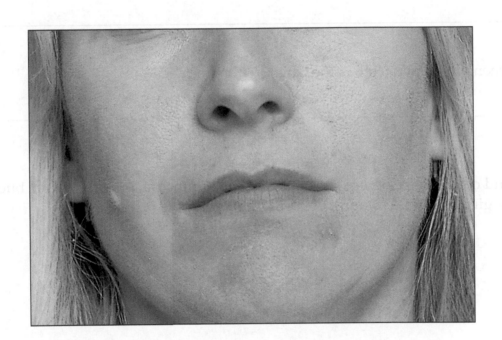

Structures of the Oral Cavity—Maxillary View

1. The deepest point of the vestibule is called the _____.

   A. labial frenum

   B. alveolar mucosa

   C. gingiva

   D. vestibule fornix

2. Name, in order, the landmarks starting up from the maxillary central enamel surface.

   _____

3. Between which two teeth is the labial frenum located?

   _____

Label and color the following landmarks: alveolar mucosa, buccal frenum, buccal mucosa, gingiva, labial frenum, vestibule, and vestibule fornix.

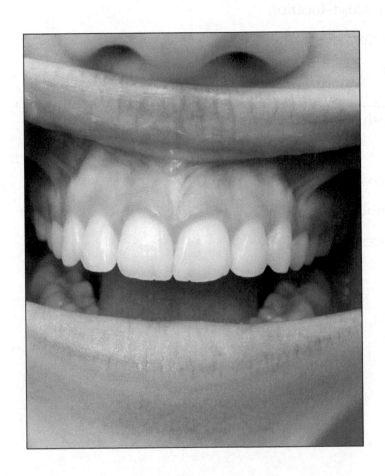

Structures of the Oral Cavity—Mandibular View

Label and color the following landmarks: alveolar mucosa, gingiva, and labial mucosa.

1. The mucosa is the tissue that lines the inner surface of the _____ and it is named according to _____.

    A. lips and cheeks–location

    B. alveolar mucosa–location

    C. gingiva–color

    D. lips–color

2. The _____ is/are loosely attached and is/are highly vascular, giving this tissue a reddish color.

    A. gingiva

    B. labial mucosa

    C. alveolar mucosa

    D. commissures

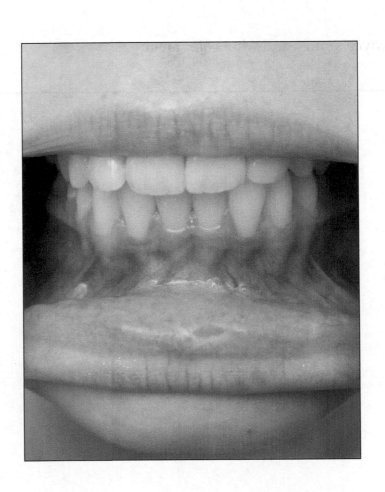

Landmark on the Buccal Mucosa

Label and color the linea alba.

Label and draw in "Fordyce's spots."

1. Describe linea alba and where it is found.

   _____

2. What are Fordyce's spots and what color are they?

   _____

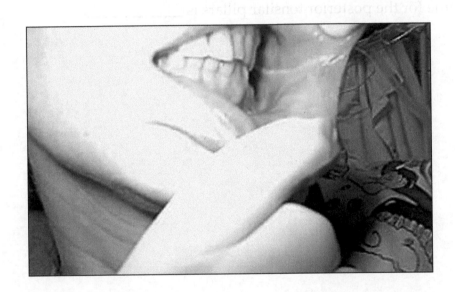

Landmarks of the Oral Pharynx Area

Label and color the following landmarks: anterior tonsiliar pillar, fauces, palatine tonsils, posterior tonsilar pillar.

Mix and match:

1. _____ fauces

A. projection extending from the back of the soft palate

2. _____ palatine tonsils

B. space in the back of the oral cavity

3. _____ uvula

C. located between two set of pillars

Another name for the posterior tonsilar pillars is _____.

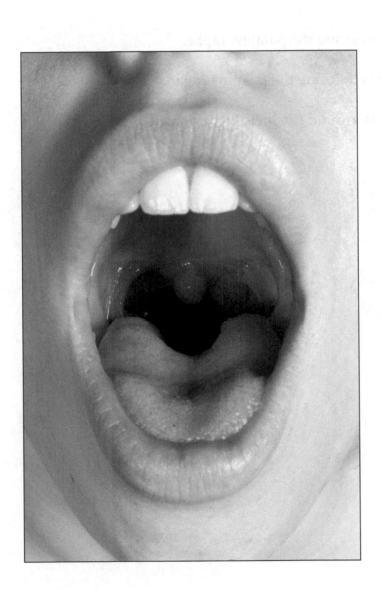

Landmarks of the Palate

1. The line that extends down the middle of the hard palate is the _____.

2. The raised area just behind the maxillary central incisors is the _____.

3. The raised horizontal lines found on the palate are the _____.

Draw a red line to locate the palatine raphe.

Draw yellow lines to locate the palatine rugae.

Draw a blue circle around the incisive papilla.

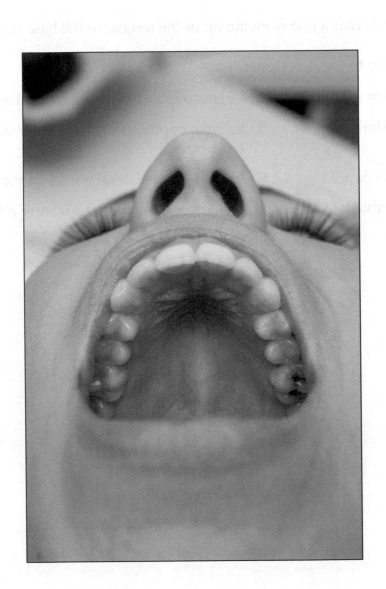

Landmarks on the Dorsal Surface of the Tongue

Label and color the following papillae: circumvallate, filiform, foliate, and fungiform.

The tongue is divided in half by the _____.

Label, draw, and color a line from the tip of the tongue to the base of the tongue.

Match the papilla to the description.

1. _____ filiform papilla

2. _____ fungiform papilla

3. _____ foliate papilla

4. _____ circumvallate papilla

A. largest papilla and mushroom shaped

B. hairlike papilla covering the dorsal side of the tongue

C. located on the lateral border of the tongue

D. give the tongue the "strawberry effect"

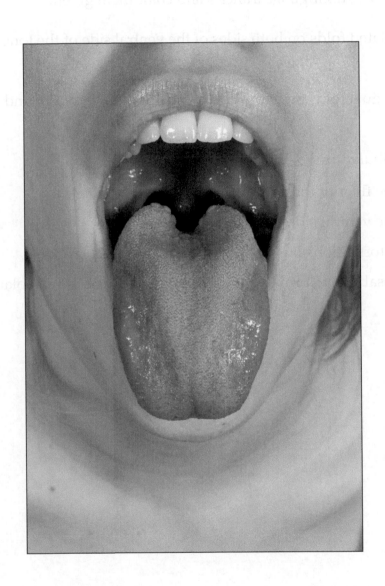

Landmarks on the Ventral Surface of the Tongue

Label the lingual frenum and color it red.

Label the lingual vein and color it blue.

Label and color the sublingual caruncles and color them green.

Label the fimbriated folds on both sides of the ventral side of the tongue and shade them yellow.

Label the sublingual folds on both sides of the floor of the mouth and shade them pink.

Describe mandibular tori: _____

A. glands on the floor of the mouth

B. glands on the ventral sides of the tongue

C. excess bone formations on the lingual side of the alveolar bone

D. excess mucosal tissue formations on the lingual side of the alveolar bone

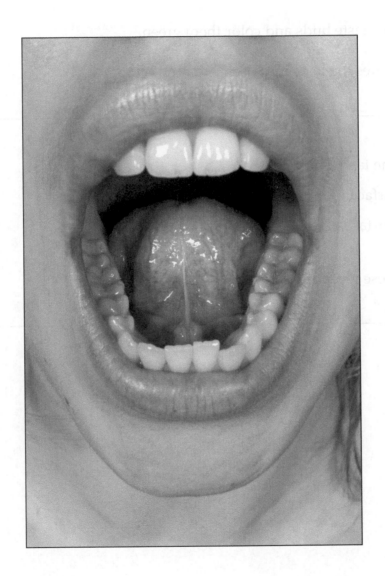

Basic Taste Buds of the Tongue

Label the "sour" taste buds and color them yellow.

Label the "sweet" taste buds and color them pink.

Label the "bitter" taste buds and color them brown.

Label the "salty" taste buds and color them green.

1. What stimulates the taste impulses?

   _____

2. Where are the taste buds located?

   A. dorsal surface of the tongue

   B. ventral surface of the tongue

3. Where do these receptors carry the taste impulses to?

   _____

Salivary Glands and Ducts

1. Which gland empties directly into the mouth?

   _____

2. Which of the glands is the largest?

   _____

3. Which duct ends in the sublingual caruncles?

   _____

Label and color the parotid gland and the Stensen's duct.

Label and draw an arrow to the buccinator muscle and the masseter muscle.

Label and color the submandibular gland and the Wharton's duct.

Label and color the sublingual gland.

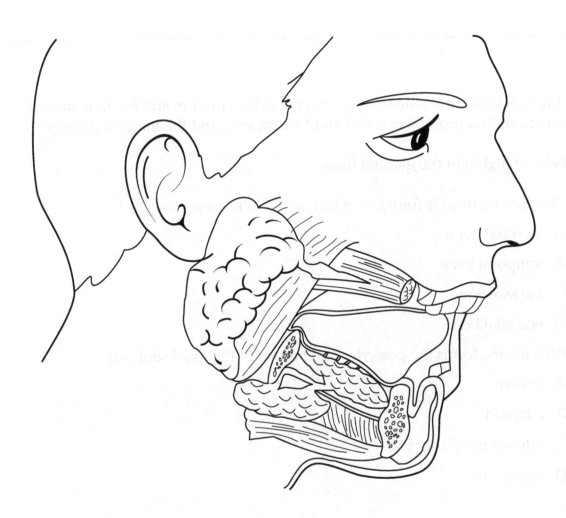

Lateral Aspect of the Cranium and Face

List, label, and then outline the bones of the cranium.

_____

List, label, and color the bones of the face that can be seen.

_____

Identify and label the following landmarks of the cranium and the face: mental foramen, styloid process, external auditory meatus, and the mastoid process.

Label and highlight the glenoid fossa.

1. The glenoid fossa is found on which of the following bones?

   A. lacrimal bone

   B. temporal bone

   C. parietal bone

   D. occipital bone

2. Which bone forms the posterior and bottom of the nasal septum?

   A. vomer

   B. ethmoid

   C. inferior nasal conchae

   D. zygomatic

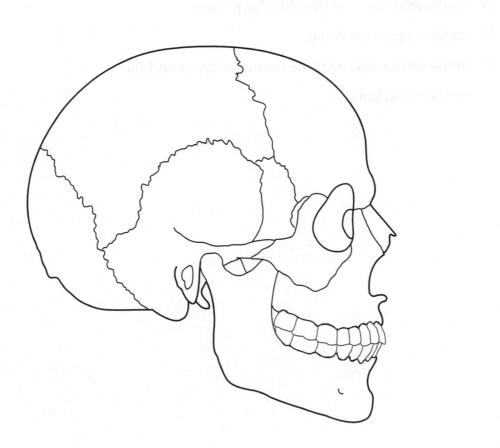

Frontal View of the Bones of the Cranium and Face

Using the same colors used in the figure on page 67, color in the bones of the face.

Label and color the inferior nasal conchae and the vomer.

Mark the alveolar process on the maxillary and mandibular.

1. Where is the symphysis found?

   A. on the maxilla near the alveolar process

   B. on the zygomatic bone

   C. in the center and near the border of the mandible

   D. on the nasal bone

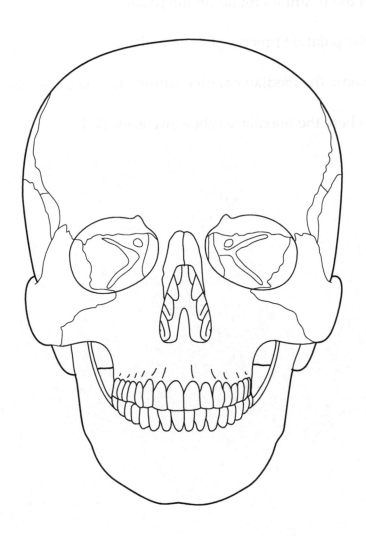

Landmarks of the Palate

How many foramina are there in total on the palate?

_____

Outline and label the foramina found on the palate.

Label and color the palatine process of the maxilla.

Draw arrows to show the median palatine suture and the transverse palatine suture.

Draw a red "X" where the maxillary tuberosity is located.

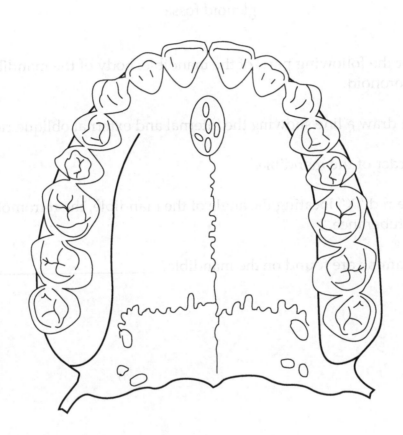

Lateral View of the External Surface of the Mandible

Mix and match:

1. _____ ramus   A. anterior portion of the ramus

2. _____ coronoid process   B. extends from the mental foramen, passes the last
                                           tooth, and curves up on the ramus

3. _____ condyle   C. the vertical portion of the mandible

4. _____ external oblique   D. the part of the mandible that articulates with the
   ridge   glenoid fossa

Label and color the following parts of the mandible: body of the mandible, ramus, condyle, and coronoid.

Label and then draw a line showing the internal and external oblique ridges.

Outline the border of the mandible.

Label and put a red "X" locating the angle of the mandible, the retromolar area, and the mental protuberance.

How many foramina are found on the mandible? _____

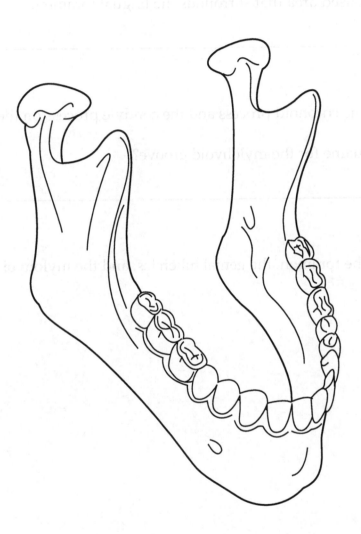

Internal Lingual View of the Mandible

List the foramina seen on the lingual side of the mandible.

_____

Name the bony raised area that surrounds the lingual foramen.

_____

Label and color the coronoid process and the condyle process on the mandible.

What is another name for the mylohyoid groove?

_____

Label and color the foramen, the genial tubercles, and the mylohyoid groove.

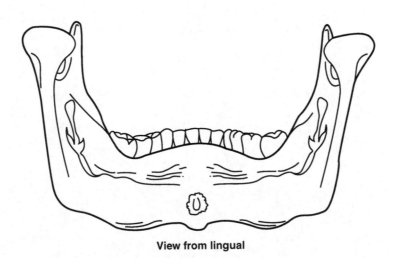

View from lingual

Temporomandibular Joint (TMJ)

What part of the mandible is part of the temporomandibular joint? Label and color.

A. coronoid

B. condyle

Label and color the glenoid fossa.

Label and color the upper and lower joint cavities.

The _____ lies between the condyle and the glenoid fossa. Label and color.

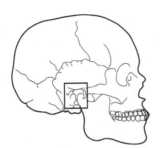

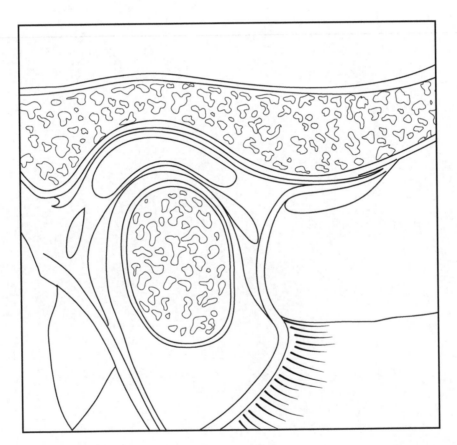

Movement of the Temporomandibular Joint (TMJ)–Hinge Joint

Label and color the articular disc.

Label and color the condyle of the mandible.

Label and color the glenoid fossa.

Another name for articular disc is the _____.

Draw a line pointing to the articular eminence.

Describe the hinge motion of the TMJ.

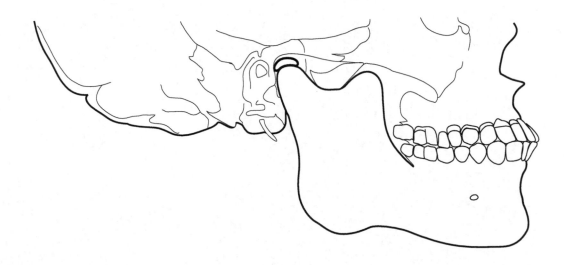

Movement of the Temporalmandibular Joint (TMJ)– Gliding Joint

Label and color the articular disc using the same color as in figure on page 79.

Label and color the condyle of the mandible using the same color as in figure on page 79.

Label and color the glenoid fossa using the same color as in figure on page 79.

Describe the gliding movement of the TMJ.

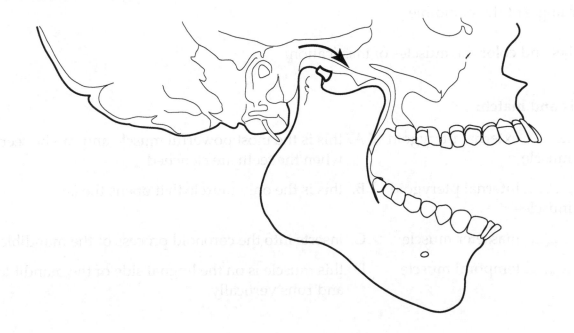

Muscles of Mastication–Lateral View

List the muscles of mastication.

_____

_____

_____

_____

Label and color the following landmarks: neck of the condyle, zygomatic bone, and the angle of the mandible.

Label and color the muscles of mastication.

Mix and match:

1. _____ external pterygoid muscle

2. _____ internal pterygoid muscle

3. _____ masseter muscle

4. _____ temporal muscle

A. this is the most powerful muscle and can be seen when the teeth are clenched

B. this is the only muscle that opens the jaw

C. inserts into the coronoid process of the mandible

D. this muscle is on the lingual side of the mandible and runs vertically

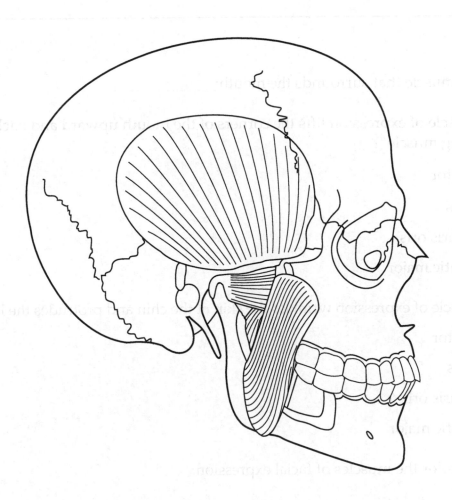

Muscles of Facial Expression

List the four main facial muscles of expression.

_____

_____

_____

_____

Name the muscle that surrounds the mouth: _____

Which muscle of expression lifts the corners of the mouth upward and backward, the "smiling muscle"?

A. buccinator

B. mentalis

C. orbicularis oris

D. zygomatic major

Which muscle of expression wrinkles the skin of the chin and protrudes the lower lip?

A. buccinator

B. mentalis

C. orbicularis oris

D. zygomatic major

Label and color the muscles of facial expression.

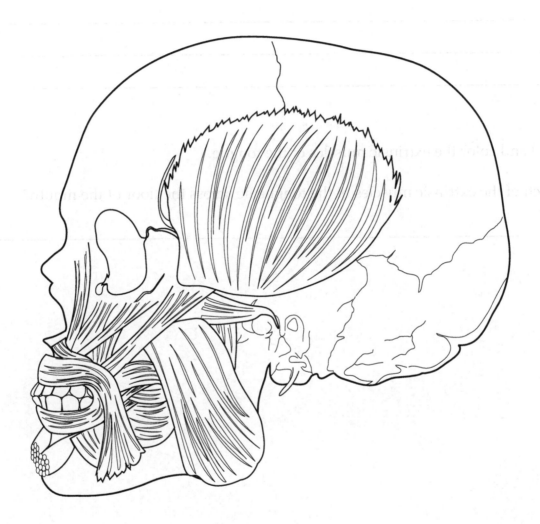

Extrinsic Muscles of the Tongue

Label and color the following landmarks: hyoid bone, styloid process, and the dorsum of the tongue.

List the extrinsic muscles of the tongue.

_____

_____

_____

_____

Label and color the extrinsic muscles of the tongue.

Which of the extrinsic muscles of the tongue lie across the floor of the mouth?

_____

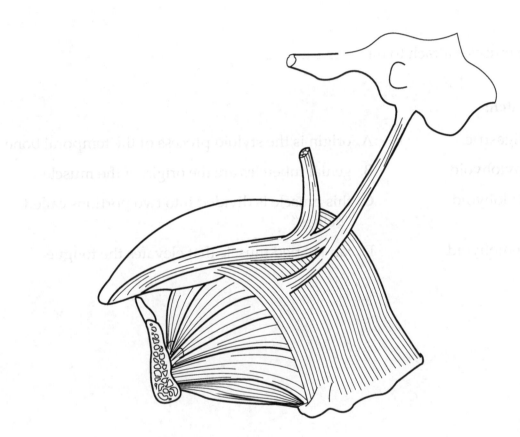

Muscles of the Floor of the Mouth

List, label, and color the muscles of the floor of the mouth.

_____

_____

_____

_____

All of these muscles attach to the _____.

Mix and match:

1. _____ digastric

2. _____ mylohyoid

3. _____ stylohyoid

4. _____ geniohyoid

A. origin is the styloid process of the temporal bone

B. genial tubercles are the origin of the muscle

C. this muscle is divided into two portions called "bellies"

D. fan-shaped muscle that elevates the tongue

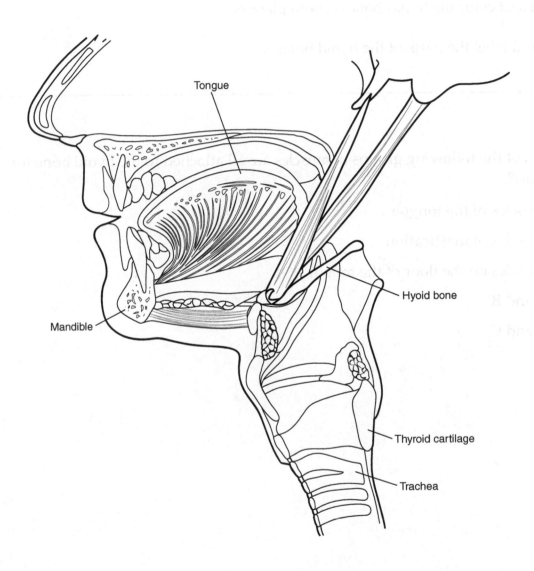

Tongue

Mandible

Hyoid bone

Thyroid cartilage

Trachea

The Hyoid Bone

The hyoid bone is located below the posterior of the _____ at the base of the tongue and in front of the _____. It is a free-floating bone for _____ to attach.

Label and color the hyoid bone on both pictures.

List and label the parts of the hyoid bone:

_____

Which of the following groups of muscles are all attached to the hyoid bone for support?

A. muscles of the tongue

B. muscles of mastication

C. muscles on the floor of the mouth

D. A and B

E. A and C

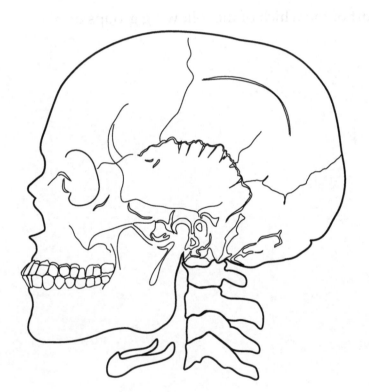

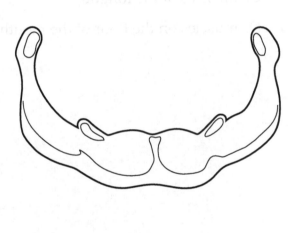

Muscles of the Soft Palate

Label and color the two muscles of the soft palate.

Draw a line to the uvula and the nasopharynx area.

What is the function of these two muscles of the soft palate?

_____

The palatoglossus muscles are also a part of the which of the following groups of muscles?

A. muscles of mastication

B. muscles of the facial expression

C. muscles of the tongue

D. muscles on the floor of the mouth

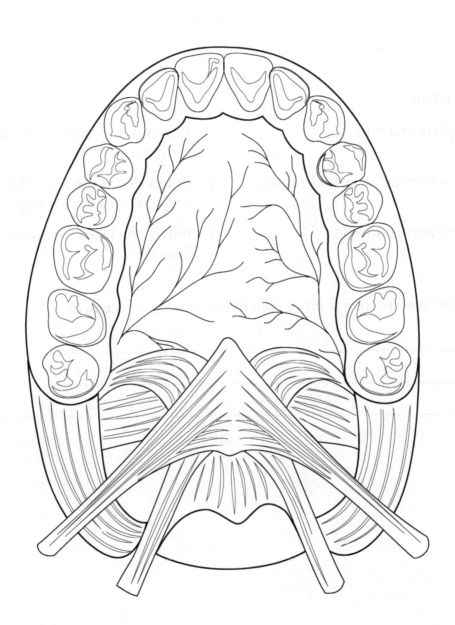

Muscles of the Neck

List, label, and color the muscles of the neck:

_____

_____

_____

Mix and match:

1. _____ platysma muscle

    A. this muscle assists in elevating the chin

2. _____ sternocleidomastoid muscle

    B. draws down the mandible, corners of the mouth, and the lip

3. _____ trapezius muscle

    C. moves the head backward and laterally

List and label the *insertion point* of each of the muscles of the neck:

_____

_____

_____

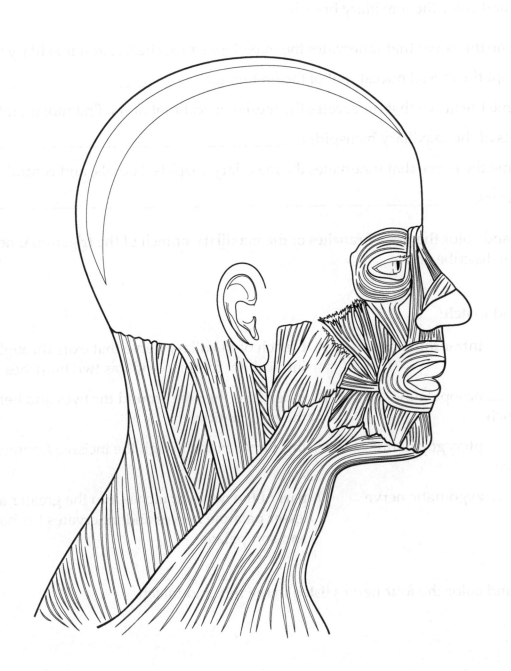

Nerves of the Maxillary Arch

Label and color the trigeminal ganglion and the pterygopalatine ganglion.

Label and color the maxillary branch.

1. Name the nerve that innervates the maxillary sinus, cheeks, and maxillary molars except the mesial buccal root of the first molar. _____

2. Name the nerve that innervates the mesial buccal root of the first molar and the roots of the maxillary bicuspids. _____

3. Name the nerve that innervates the maxillary cuspids, laterals, and central incisors. _____

Label and color the three branches of the maxillary branch of the trigeminal nerve that are describe above.

Mix and match:

1. _____ infraorbital nerve

2. _____ nasopalatine branch

3. _____ pterygopalatine nerve

4. _____ zygomatic nerve

A. branch of maxillary nerve that exits through the infraorbital foramen and has two branches

B. innervates the area around the eyes and behind the zygomatic arch

C. this nerve exits through the incisive foramen

D. part of the nerve branches into the greater and lesser palatine nerves and innervates the hard and soft palate

Label and color the four nerves listed in the mix and match.

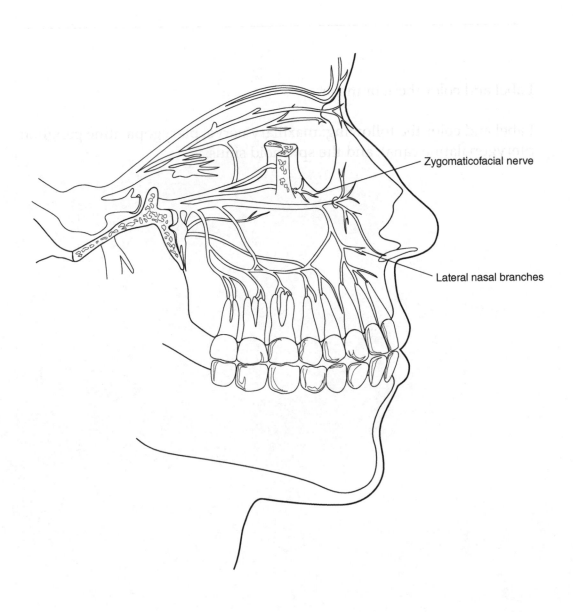

Zygomaticofacial nerve

Lateral nasal branches

Medial View of the Branches of the Pterygopalatine Nerve

List the three branches of the pterygopalatine nerve:

_____

_____

_____

Label and color these branches.

Label and color the following: maxillary nerve, pterygopalatine ganglion, pterygopalatine canal, and the sphenoid sinus.

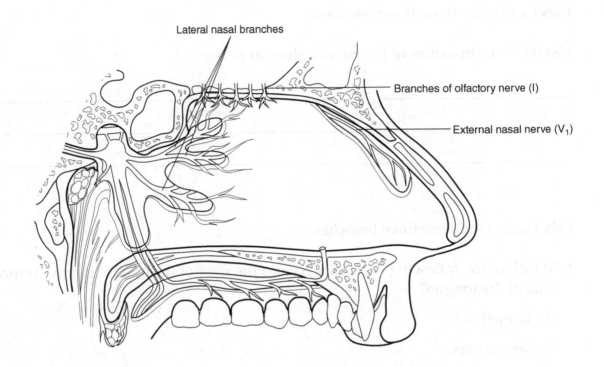

Lateral nasal branches

Branches of olfactory nerve (I)

External nasal nerve (V$_1$)

Mandibular Nerves

List the three branches of the mandibular nerve:

_____

_____

_____

Label and color these three branches.

List the three branches of the inferior alveolar nerve:

_____

_____

_____

Label and color these three branches.

1. Which of the following nerves innervates the floor of the mouth and the ventral side of the tongue?

   A. lingual nerve

   B. buccal nerve

   C. mental nerve branch

   D. none of the above

2. This nerve innervates the premolars and molars and the gingiva:

   A. buccal branch

   B. lingual branch

   C. inferior alveolar nerve branch

3. The incisive nerve branch innervates the anterior teeth and the labial gingiva:

   A. This is a true statement.

   B. This is a false statement.

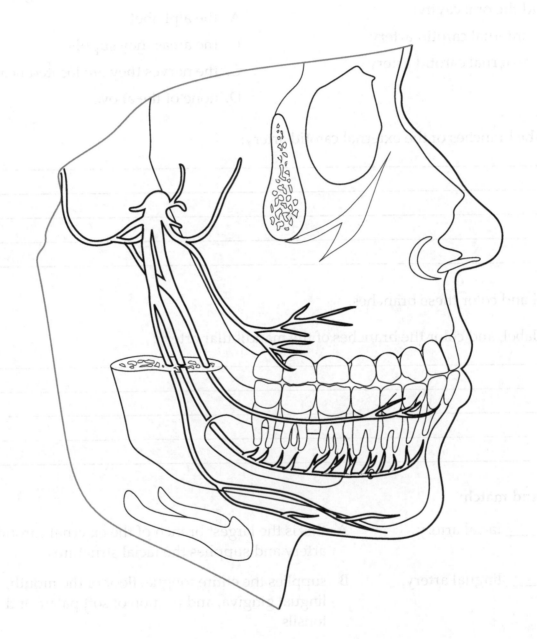

Arteries of the Face and Oral Cavity

Label the common carotid artery.

1. This artery supplies blood to the face and the oral cavity:

    A. internal carotid artery

    B. external carotid artery

2. Branches are named according to:

    A. the alphabet

    B. the areas they supply

    C. the nerves they are located near

    D. none of the above

List the branches of the external carotid artery:

_____

_____

_____

_____

_____

Label and color these branches.

List, label, and color the branches of the mandibular artery:

_____

_____

_____

_____

_____

Mix and match:

1. _____ facial artery

2. _____ lingual artery

3. _____ middle superior alveolar artery

4. _____ incisive artery

5. _____ maxillary artery

A. this is the largest branch of the external carotid artery and supplies the facial structures

B. supplies the entire tongue, floor of the mouth, lingual gingiva, and portion of soft palate and tonsils

C. this artery has six branches and branches across the mandible to the corners of the mouth, then upward toward the eye

D. supplies the maxillary premolars

E. supplies the mandibular anterior teeth

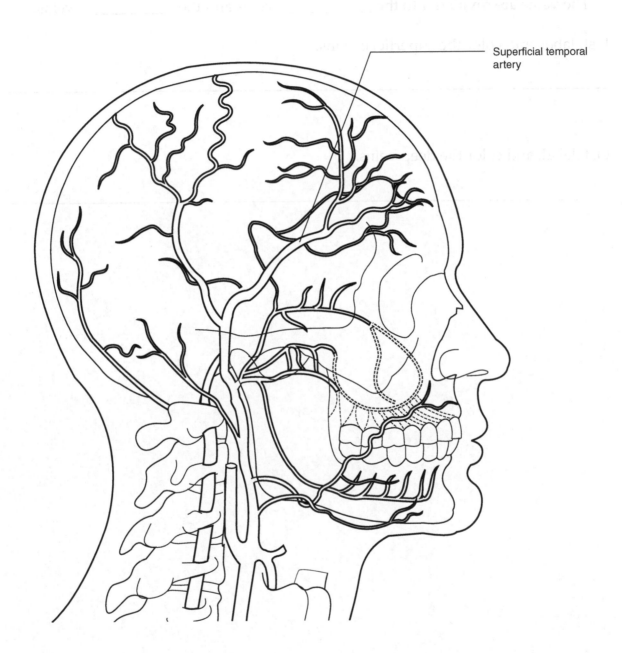

Superficial temporal
artery

Veins of the Face and Oral Cavity

1. The _____ vein drains the blood from the cranium, face, and neck into the superior vena cava.

2. The veins are divided into the _____ veins and the _____ veins.

List, label, and color the superficial veins.

_____

List, label, and color the deep veins.

_____

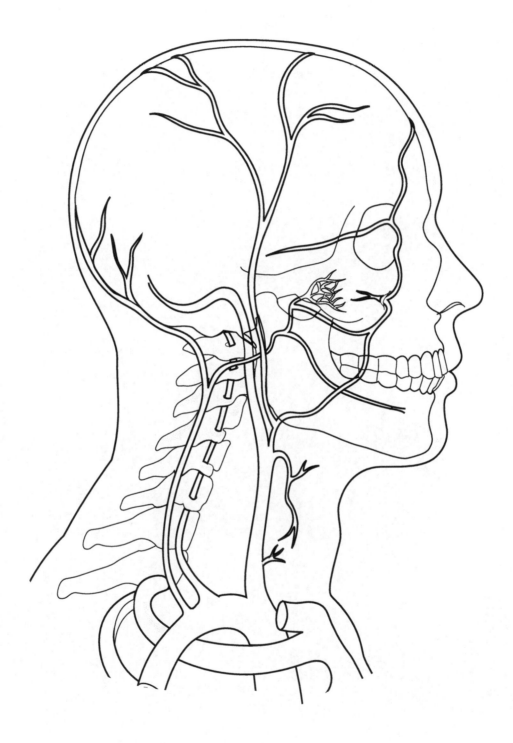

Tooth and Tissue Structures

The Three Primary Embryonic Layers

Match the structure to the definition. Label and color the structure on the illustration and write the names of at least four tissues in each colored area that are differentiated from this primary embryonic layer.

1. _____ mesoderm
2. _____ endoderm
3. _____ ectoderm

A. the outer embryonic layer
B. the middle embryonic layer
C. the inner embryonic layer

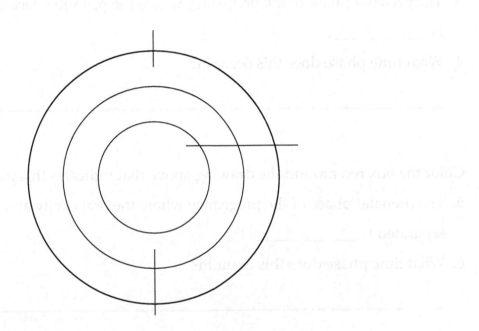

Embryology

1. The prenatal phase of the pregnancy where rapid cell division and differentiation occurs is _____.

2. In what time phase does this occur?

   _____

Color the box blue around the drawing above that indicates this phase.

3. The prenatal phase of the pregnancy where the primitive face develops is _____.

4. What time phase does this occur in?

   _____

Color the box red around the drawing above that indicates this phase.

5. The prenatal phase of the pregnancy where the oral cavity and nasal cavity are separated is _____.

6. What time phase does this occur in?

   _____

Color the box green around the drawing above that indicates this phase.

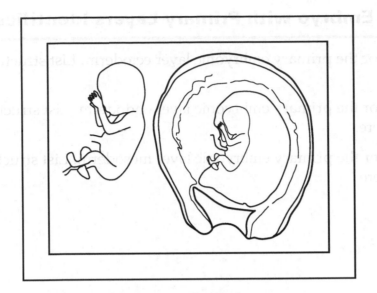

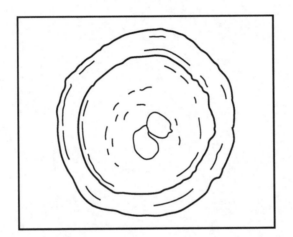

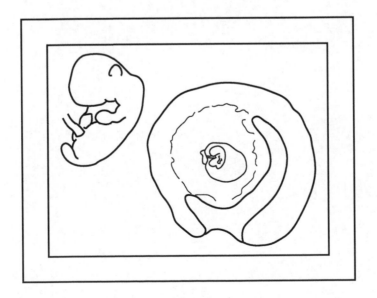

Developing Embryo with Primary Layers Identified

1. Label and color the primary embryonic layer ectoderm. List structures you would find here.

2. Label and color the primary embryonic layer endoderm. List structures you would find here.

3. Label and color the primary embryonic layer mesoderm. List structures you would find here.

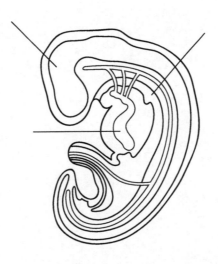

Facial Processes Shown on an Embryo (Child and Adult)

Identify and color the mandibular process red on the embryo, child, and adult line drawings.

Identify and color the philtrum blue on the adult and child line drawings.

Identify and color the maxillary process green on the adult, child, and embryo line drawings.

Identify and color the frontal process yellow on the adult, child, and embryo line drawings.

Identify and place a black star on the labial commissures on the adult and child line drawings.

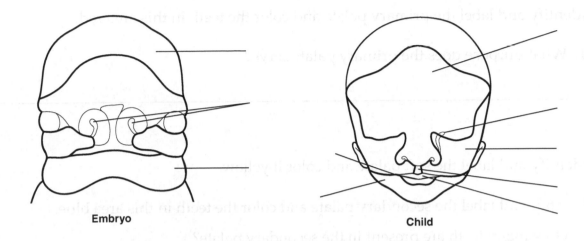

Embryo   **Child**

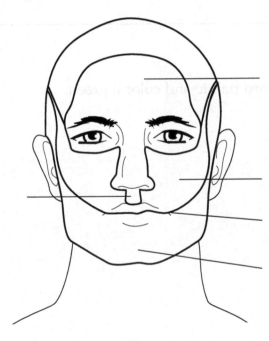

Adult

Development of the Palate

Draw a black line to identify the median palatine suture and the incisive suture.

Identify and label the primary palate and color the teeth in this area red.

1. What purpose does the primary palate serve?

_____

Identify and label the soft palate and color it yellow.

Identify and label the secondary palate and color the teeth in this area blue.

2. How many teeth are present in the secondary palate?

_____

Identify and label the hard palate and color it green.

Bilateral Cleft of the Lip (Alveolar Process and Primary Palate)

Label and color the following structures: palatine rugae, incisive papilla, median palatine raphe, hard palate, alveolar process, lips, uvula, and soft palate. Answer the following questions:

1. How many teeth types are seen in this figure?

2. Are the lips, nor central areas lost or not?

3. How many uvulae (1) palate is cut?

4. The cleft palate is running along the incisive canal until bone is seen?

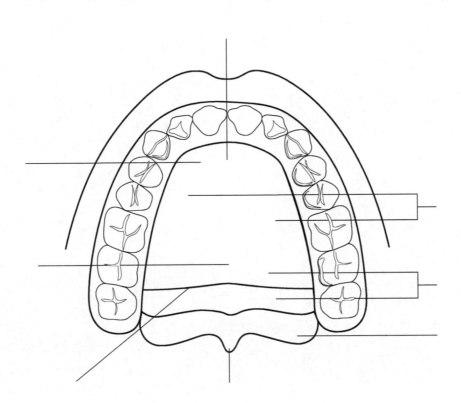

Bilateral Cleft of the Lip (Alveolar Process and Primary Palate)

Label and color the following: secondary palate, primary palate, philtrum, hard and soft palate, alveolar process, lip, uvula, incisive papillae.

1. How many cleft lips occur in 1,000 live births? _____

2. Are cleft lips more common in boys or girls? _____

3. How many cleft palates occur? _____

4. Are cleft palates occurring alone more common in boys or girls? _____.

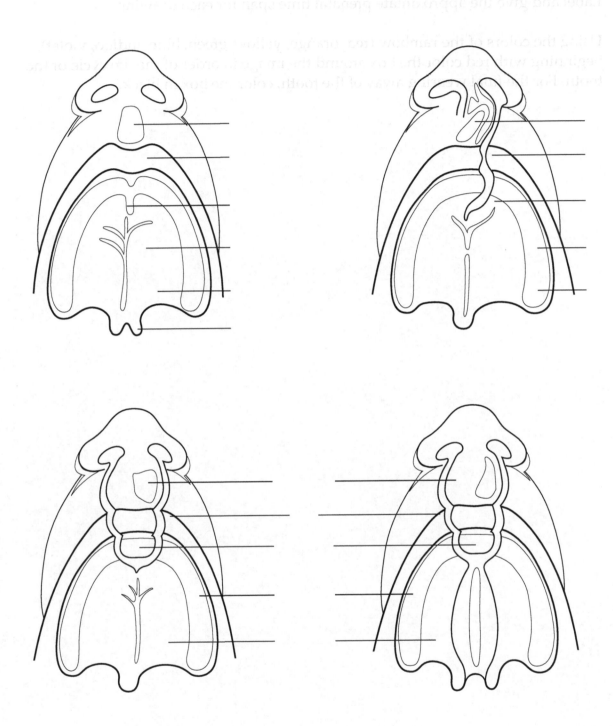

Life Cycle of the Tooth

Label and give the approximate prenatal time span for each drawing.

Using the colors of the rainbow (red, orange, yellow, green, blue, indigo, violet), beginning with red color the box around the image in order of the life cycle of the tooth. For the final wearing away of the tooth, color the box in black.

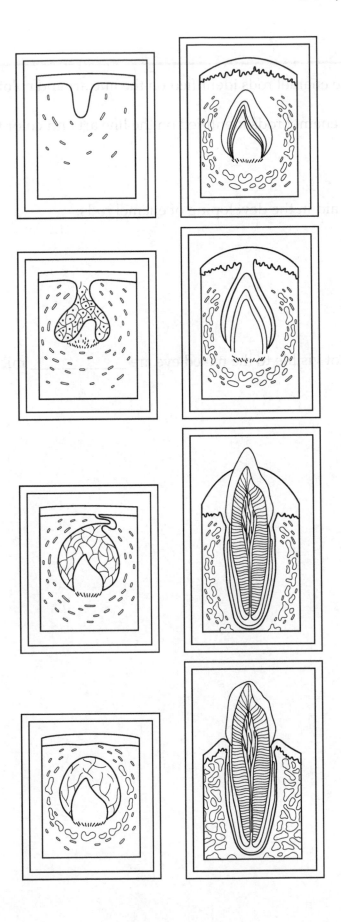

Enamel Rods

Label the heads of the enamel rods identified on the line art and color them red.

Label the tales of the enamel rods identified on the line art and color them blue.

Multiple choice:

1. The _____ aid in the developing of enamel rods.

   A. cementoblasts

   B. odontoblasts

   C. ameloblasts

   D. pulpoblasts

2. The enamel rods not visible to the naked eye are _____ micrometers in diameter.

   A. 6

   B. 4

   C. 10

   D. 2

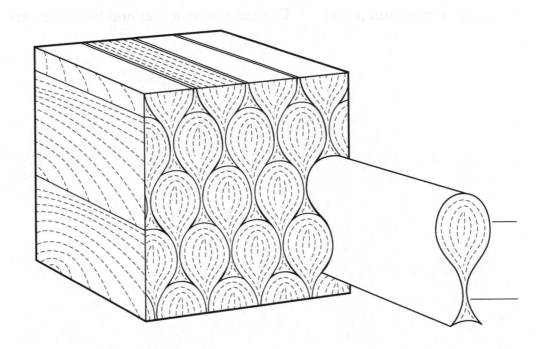

Tissues of the Tooth

Match, color, and label the following tissues of the tooth:

1. _____ enamel (green)

2. _____ dentin (yellow)

3. _____ pulp (red)

4. _____ cementum (blue)

A. the structure located around the root, it covers the dentin on the root portion of the tooth

B. the hardest living tissue in the body

C. makes up the bulk of the tooth

D. made from nerves and blood vessels

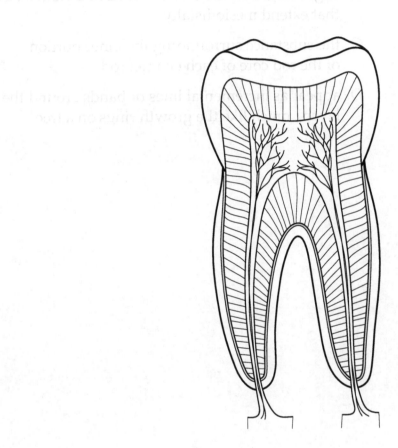

Enamel

Locate and color the enamel on the line art.

Mix and match:

1. _____ lines of Retzius

   A. accentuated incremental lines that indicate the trauma of birth

2. _____ interprismatic substance

   B. slight ridges on the cervical third of certain teeth that extend mesiodistally

3. _____ neonatal line

   C. the substance surrounding the inner portion of the rod core of each enamel rod

4. _____ imbrication lines

   D. appear as incremental lines or bands around the layers, much like the growth rings on a tree

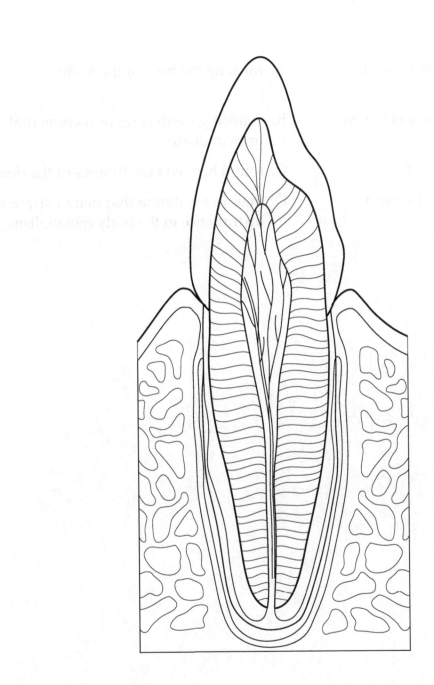

Dentin

Locate and color the dentin on the line art.

Mix and match:

1. _____ imbrication lines of Von Ebner

2. _____ contour lines of Owen

3. _____ primary dentin

4. _____ intertubular dentin

A. forming the bulk of the tooth

B. stained growth rings or incremental lines in dentin

C. found between the tubules of the dentin

D. lines in the dentin that demonstrate a disturbance in the body metabolism

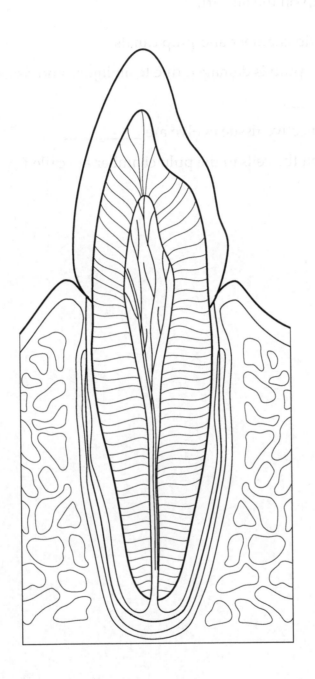

Pulp

Locate and color the pulp on the line art.

Label the pulp horns, pulp chamber and pulp canals.

1. A condition where the pulp is damaged due to an injury and tissue becomes inflamed is _____.

2. Cells from which connective tissue evolve are _____.

3. The substance between the cells in the pulp chamber are called _____.

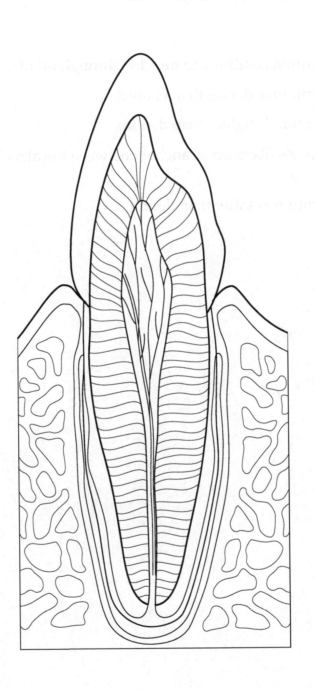

Cementum

Locate and color the cementum on the line art.

True or false:

1. _____ the cementum continues to develop throughout life.

2. _____ the cementum is darker than enamel.

3. _____ the cementum is lighter than dentin.

4. _____ the Sharpey's fibers act as anchors between the alveolar bone and the dentin.

5. _____ the cementum is softer than dentin.

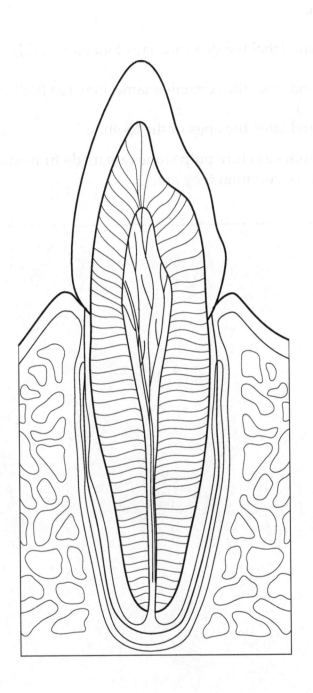

Tooth and Surrounding Tissues

Label and color the pulp, cementum, lamina dura, gingival tissue, alveolar process, dentin, and enamel.

Draw an arrow to and label the dentinoenamel junction (DEJ).

Draw an arrow to and label the cementoenamel junction (CEJ).

Draw an arrow to and label the apex of the tooth.

1. Describe what tooth structure pulp stones are made from and discuss where they are located and how common they are.

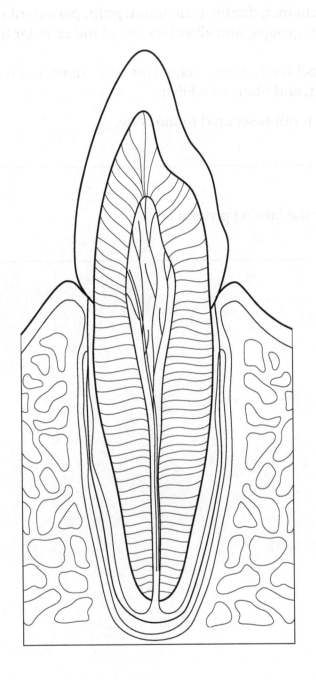

Sharpey's Fibers and Cementum

Label and color the enamel, dentin, cementum, pulp, periodontal ligaments, lamina propria gingival fiber groups, and alveolar crest of the alveolar bone proper.

Draw arrows and label the cementoenamel junction, dentinocementum junction, epithelial attachment, and Sharpey's Fibers.

1. Describe how the tooth is secured to the bone.

    _____

2. Another name for the lamina propria is

    _____

.

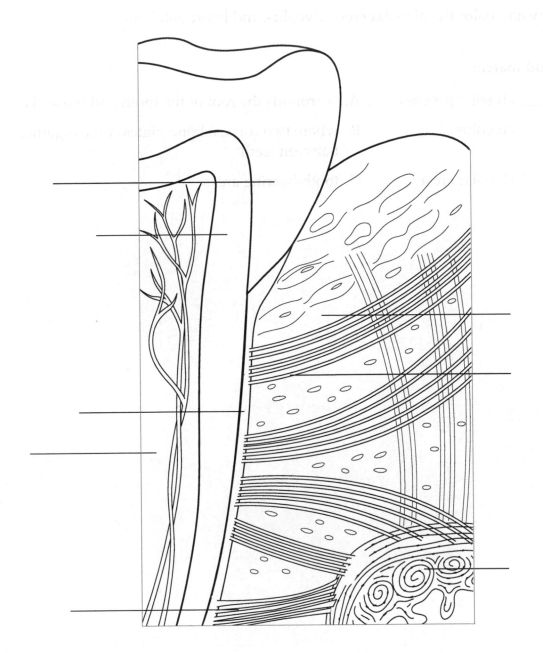

Periodontal Ligaments and Alveolar Crests

Identify and color the alveolar crest, alveolus, and interdental bone.

Mix and match:

1. _____ alveolar process
2. _____ alveolus
3. _____ alveolar crest

A. surrounds the root of the tooth and the socket

B. where two cortical bone plates come together between teeth

C. tooth-bearing areas

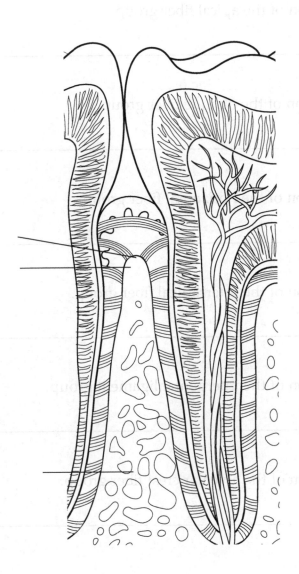

Cross Section of Mandibular Molar Tissues of the Tooth Identified

Label and color the following periodontal fiber groups: apical fiber group, horizontal fiber group, interradical septum, oblique fiber group, interdental fiber groups, and alveolar crest fiber group.

1. Describe the function of the apical fiber group.

   _____

2. Describe the function of the oblique fiber group.

   _____

3. Describe the function of the horizontal fiber group.

   _____

4. Describe the function of the interradical fiber group.

   _____

5. Describe the function of the interdental ligament group.

   _____

6. Describe the function of the alveolar crest fiber group.

   _____

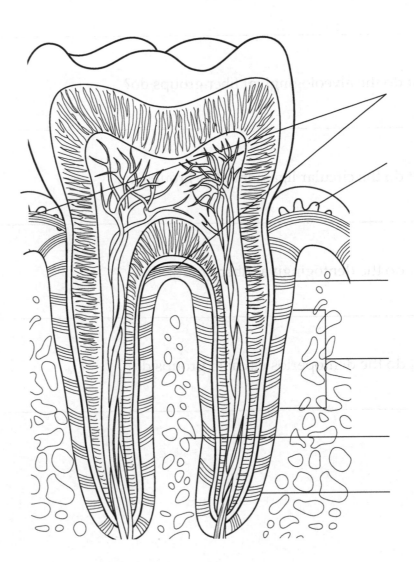

Gingival Fiber Groups

Label and color the four gingival fiber groups on the line art.

1. Where are the gingival fiber groups found?

   _____

2. What do the alveologingival fiber groups do?

   _____

3. What do the circular ligament fiber groups do?

   _____

4. What do the dentogingival fiber groups do?

   _____

5. What do the dentoperiosteal fiber groups do?

   _____

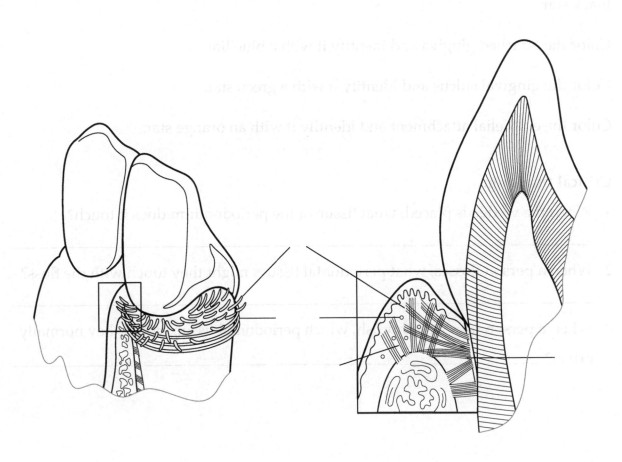

Periodontium

Identify the alveolar bone and color it tan.

Color the gingival crest and identify it with a red star.

Color the marginal gingiva and identify it with a yellow line.

Identify the mucogingival junction by drawing a line and marking the spot with a black star.

Color the attached gingiva and identify it with a blue line.

Color the gingival sulcus and identify it with a green star.

Color the epithelial attachment and identify it with an orange star.

Critical thinking:

1. When the wedge is placed, what tissue of the periodontium does it touch?

   _____

2. When a person flosses, what periodontal tissues might they touch with the floss?

   _____

3. When a person uses a toothbrush, which periodontal tissue would they normally

   brush? _____

Alveolar Mucosa

Identify the following on the line art: gingival groove, marginal gingiva, alveolar mucosa, interdental gingiva, attached gingiva, mucogingival junction. Color each of these gingival tissues on the photo.

Fill in the words (related to the periodontium):

1. _____ extends from the mucogingival junction to the gingival groove.

2. _____ is an extension of unattached gingiva between adjacent teeth.

3. _____ is the gingiva in the floor of the gingival sulcus.

4. _____ is the line of demarcation between the attached gingiva and the alveolar mucosa.

5. _____ is the line of demarcation between the attached gingiva and the marginal gingiva.

6. _____ is the space between the unattached gingiva and the tooth.

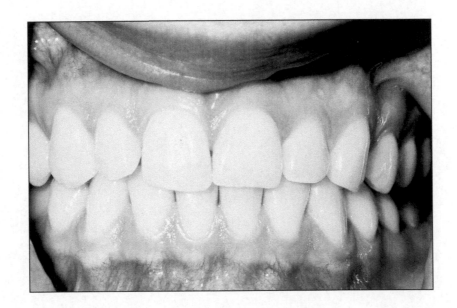

Tooth Anatomy

Adult Dentition

Draw a black line indicating the midline (median line) on the dentition.

Label the second bicuspids (premolars) and color them green.

Label the first molars and color them red.

Label the central incisors and color them yellow.

Label the cuspids (canines) and color them orange.

Label the first bicuspids (premolars) and color them blue.

Label the third molars and color them purple.

Label the lateral incisors and color them pink.

Label the second molars and color them grey.

Maxillary

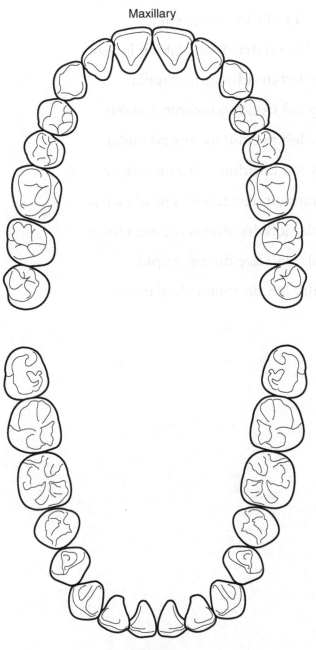

Mandibular

(A) Permanent dentition

Deciduous Dentition

Match the name of the tooth to the letter shown on the diagram. Label and color the tooth on the illustration.

1. _____ maxillary left deciduous cuspid

2. _____ mandibular left deciduous lateral incisor

3. _____ maxillary left deciduous first molar

4. _____ maxillary left deciduous central incisor

5. _____ maxillary left deciduous second molar

6. _____ maxillary left deciduous lateral incisor

7. _____ mandibular left deciduous central incisor

8. _____ mandibular left deciduous second molar

9. _____ mandibular left deciduous cuspid

10. _____ mandibular left deciduous first molar

Maxillary

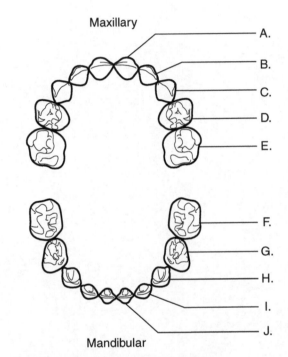

A.

B.

C.

D.

E.

F.

G.

H.

I.

J.

Mandibular

(B) Primary (deciduous) dentition

Primary Dentition

Draw the midline. (Recall that the midline is the imagery line that divides the dental arches into two halves.)

Draw a line that divides the dentition into two arches, creating four quadrants that have the same arrangement of teeth in each quadrant.

Color each of the similar teeth the same color in each quadrant.

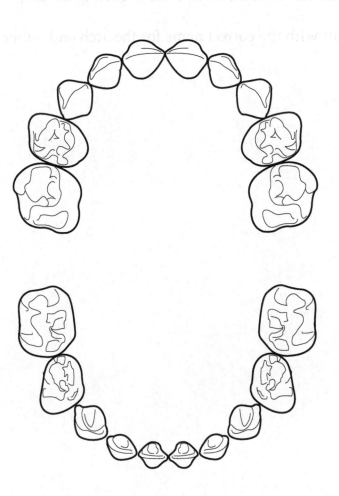

Permanent Dentition

Draw the midline. (Recall that the midline is the imagery line that divides the dental arches into two halves.)

Draw a line that divides the dentition into two arches, creating four quadrants that have the same arrangement of teeth in each quadrant.

Color each of the similar teeth the same color in each quadrant.

Label each quadrant with the correct name for the arch and either right or left.

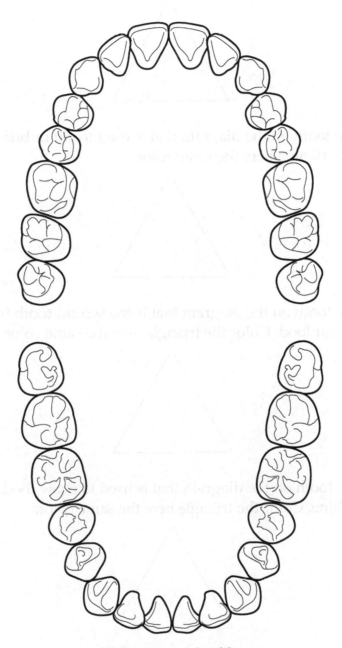

(A) Permanent dentition

Primary Teeth

Label and color the tooth on the diagram that is slightly more bulky in size and aids in tearing food. Color the triangle here the same color.

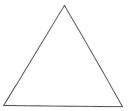

Label and color the tooth on the diagram that is used to cut or bite the food that is ingested. Color the triangle here the same color.

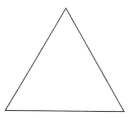

Label and color the tooth on the diagram that is the second tooth from the midline and is also used to cut food. Color the triangle here the same color.

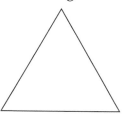

Label and color the tooth on the diagram that is used to chew food and is furthest away from the midline. Color the triangle here the same color.

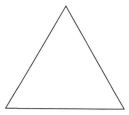

Label and color the tooth on the diagram that is used to chew food and is closer to the midline than the other one it closely resembles. Color the triangle here the same color.

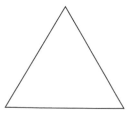

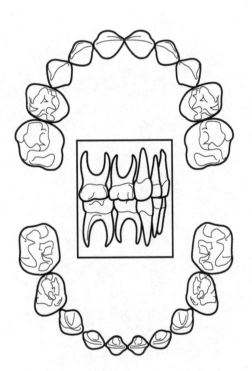

Permanent Dentition

Color each of the anterior teeth on the diagram on the following page in one color.

Identify that color here. _____

Color each of the posterior teeth on the diagram on the following page in another color.

Identify that color here. _____

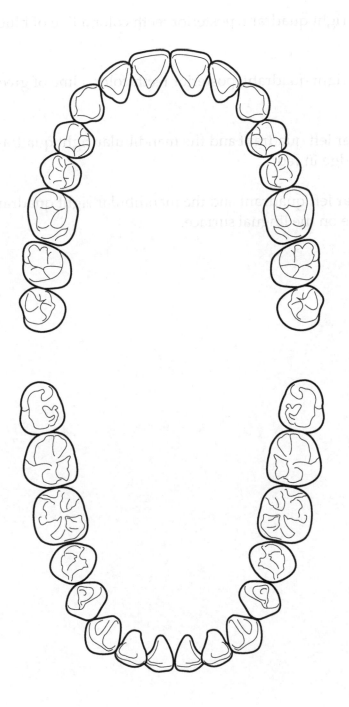

Permanent Dentition

On the maxillary right quadrant, posterior teeth color a line of red on the buccal side.

On the maxillary right quadrant, posterior teeth color a line of blue on the occlusal surface.

On the maxillary right quadrant, posterior teeth color a line of green on the lingual surface.

On the mandibular left quadrant and the mandibular right quadrant, anterior teeth color the incisal edge in red.

On the mandibular left quadrant and the mandibular right quadrant, anterior teeth color a line of blue on the lingual surface.

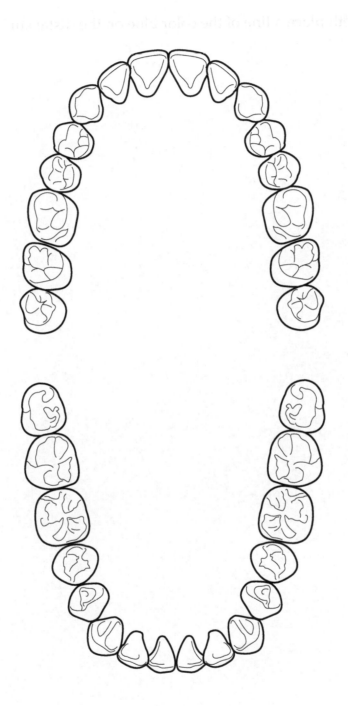

Permanent Dentition

On each of the teeth place a line of the color red on the mesial surface.

On each of the teeth place a line of the color blue on the distal surface.

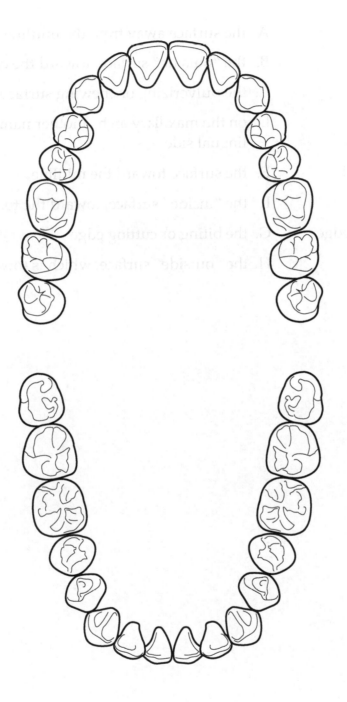

Permanent Dentition

Match the tooth surface to the definition. Label and color the surface on the illustration.

1. _____ mesial

2. _____ distal

3. _____ lingual

4. _____ buccal

5. _____ occlusal

6. _____ labial

7. _____ incisal edge

8. _____ palatal

A. the surface away from the midline

B. the "outside" surface, toward the cheek

C. the pulverizing or chewing surface

D. on the maxillary arch, another name for the lingual side

E. the surface toward the midline

F. the "inside" surface, toward the tongue

G. the biting or cutting edge

H. the "outside" surface, which is toward the lips

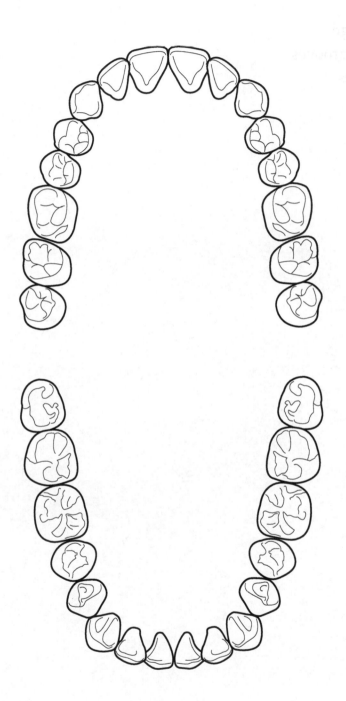

Anatomical Structures

Label and color the following landmarks on the illustration of the mandibular second molar:

- Transverse ridge
- Supplemental grooves
- Marginal ridges
- Fissure

Mandibular second molar

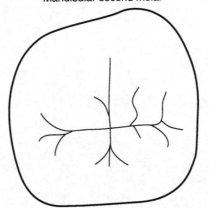

Anatomical Landmarks

Label and color the following anatomical landmarks on the correct teeth:

- Mamelons
- Cusp of Carabelli
- Oblique ridge
- Bifurcated roots

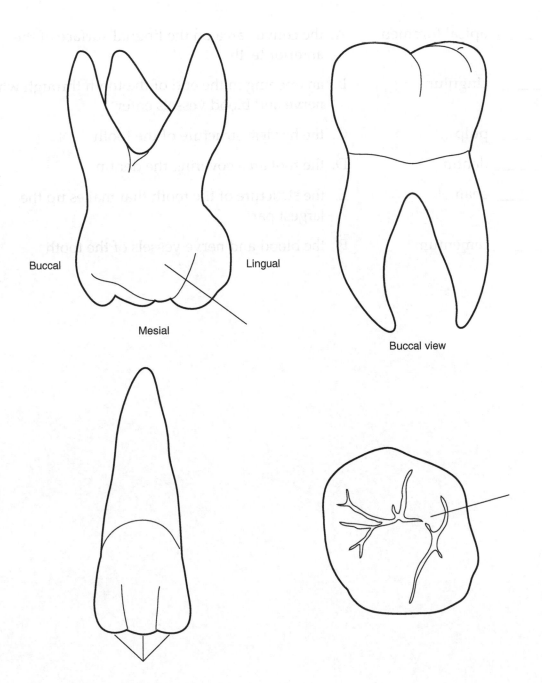

Buccal

Lingual

Mesial

Buccal view

Anatomical Landmarks

Match the structure to the definition. Label and color the structure on the illustration.

1. _____ apical foramen

   A. the convex area on the lingual surface of the anterior teeth

2. _____ cingulum

   B. an opening in the end of the tooth through which nerve and blood vessels enter

3. _____ pulp

   C. the hardest structure of the tooth

4. _____ dentin

   D. the root area covering the dentin

5. _____ enamel

   E. the structure of the tooth that makes up the largest part

6. _____ cementum

   F. the blood and nerve vessels of the tooth

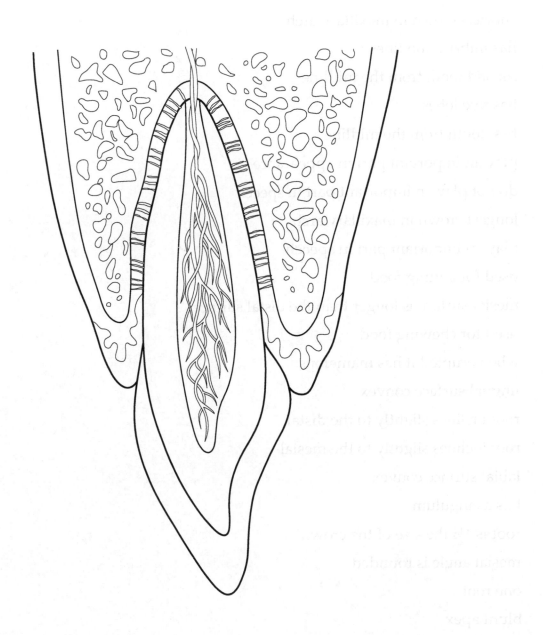

Maxillary Central Incisors

Label and color the maxillary central incisors.

Circle all that apply for the central incisor:

shortest crown in maxillary arch

has imbrication lines

second tooth from the midline

has five lobes

first tooth from the midline

play an important part in appearance

do not play an important part in speech

longest crown in maxillary arch

play an important part in speech

used for cutting food

mesial surface is longer than the distal surface

used for chewing food

when erupted it has mamelons

lingual surface convex

root inclines slightly to the distal

root inclines slightly to the mesial

labial surface convex

has a cingulum

root is 1½ the size of the crown

mesial angle is rounded

one root

blunt apex

does not have a cingulum

distal surface is longer than the mesial surface

mesial angle is acute

root is as long as the crown

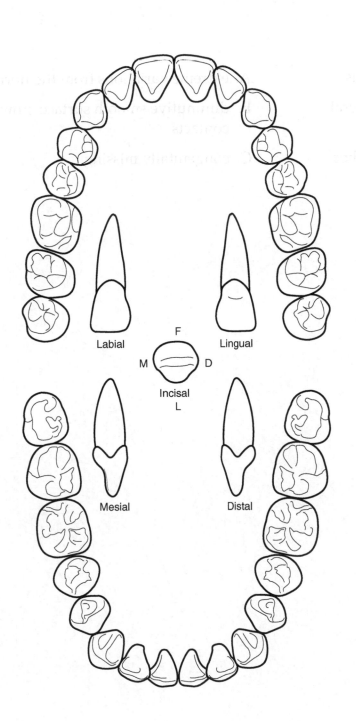

Labial

Lingual

F

M   D

Incisal

L

Mesial

Distal

Maxillary Lateral Incisors

Label and color the maxillary lateral incisors.

Mix and match:

1. _____ agenesis

A. extreme variations from the norm

2. _____ peg lateral

B. diminutive smooth surface crown lacking contacts

3. _____ anomalies

C. congenitally missing

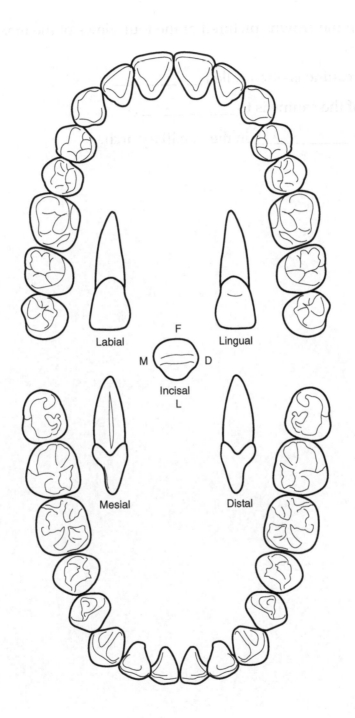

Labial

Lingual

F

M D

Incisal

L

Mesial

Distal

Maxillary Canine

Label and color the maxillary canines.

Draw the roots on the crowns pictured of the four views of the maxillary canine. Color these views.

1. The maxillary canine is often called _____.

2. The purpose of the canine is to _____.

3. The root is the _____ in the maxillary arch.

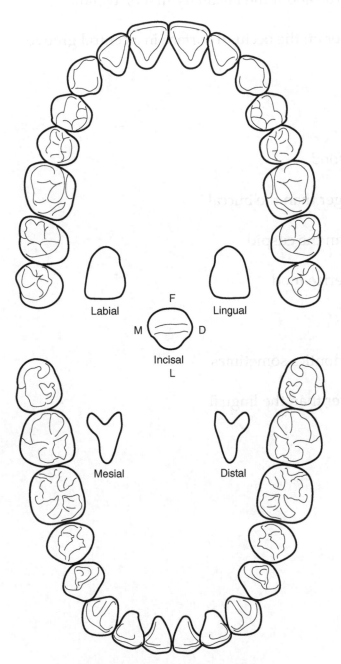

Maxillary canines (cuspids)

Maxillary First Bicuspid (Premolar)

Label and color the maxillary first bicuspid.

Circle all that are true about the maxillary first bicuspid:

cusps come together on the occlusal surface in a central groove

it is bifurcated

posterior tooth

function is to tear food

lingual cusp is longer than the buccal

roots are longer than the cuspid

function is to pulverize food

anterior tooth

removed for orthodontics sometimes

buccal cusp is longer than the lingual

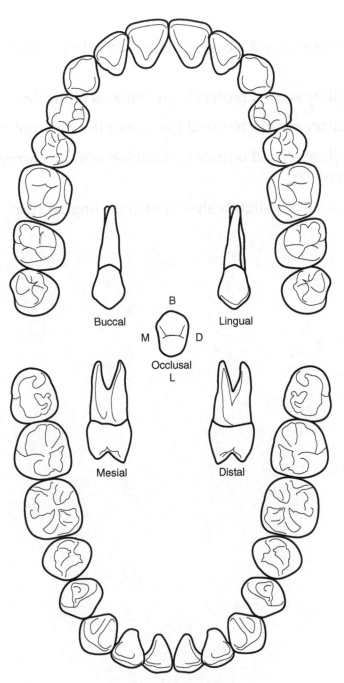

B

Buccal   Lingual

M   D

Occlusal

L

Mesial   Distal

Maxillary first premolars

Maxillary Second Bicuspid (Premolar)

Label and color the maxillary second bicuspids (premolars).

True or false:

1. _____ the maxillary second bicuspid (premolar) is larger than the first bicuspid (premolar).

2. _____ the maxillary second bicuspid (premolar) is bifurcated.

3. _____ the maxillary second bicuspid (premolar) has two root canals.

4. _____ the maxillary second bicuspid (premolar) is more narrow mesial-distally than the first premolar.

5. _____ the buccal cusp is slightly shorter than the lingual cusp.

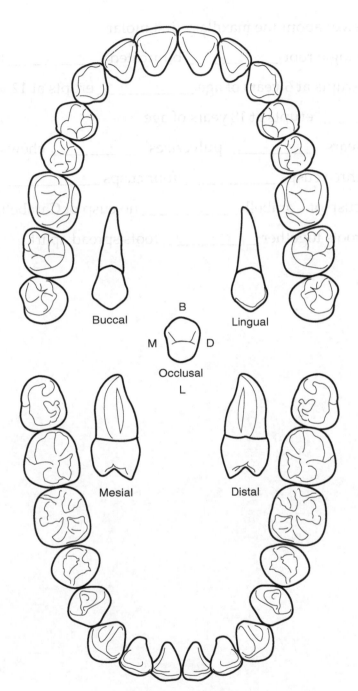

Buccal

Lingual

B

M D

Occlusal

L

Mesial

Distal

Maxillary second premolars

Maxillary First Molar

Label and color the maxillary first molar.

Mark the best answer about the maxillary first molar.

1. _____ single root _____ bifurcated _____ trifurcated

2. _____ erupts at 6 years of age _____ erupts at 12 years of age _____ erupts at 18 years of age

3. _____ tears _____ pulverizes _____ chews

4. _____ three cusps _____ four cusps _____ five cusps

5. _____ cusp of Carabelli _____ no cusp of Carabelli

6. _____ roots together _____ roots spread apart

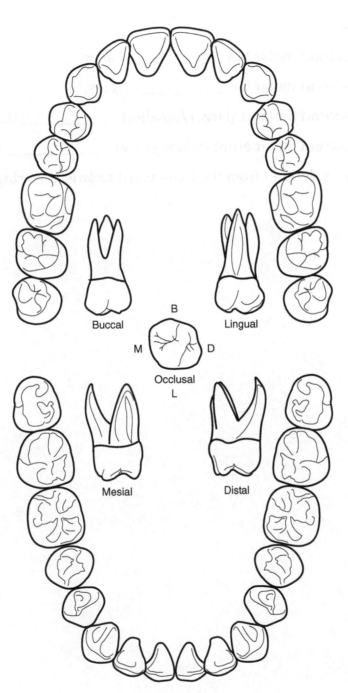

Buccal

Lingual

B

M   D

Occlusal

L

Mesial

Distal

Maxillary first molars

Maxillary Second Molar

Label and color the maxillary second molar.

Fill in the blanks:

1. The maxillary second molar has _____ cusps.

2. The maxillary second molar has _____ roots.

3. The maxillary second molar is (larger/smaller) _____ than the first molar.

4. The maxillary second molar erupts when you are _____ years of age.

5. The word molar is derived from the Latin word *molaris*, referring to a

    _____.

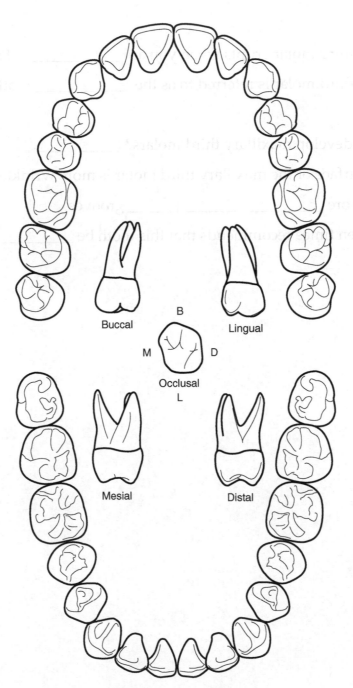

Buccal

Lingual

B

M   D

Occlusal

L

Mesial

Distal

Maxillary second molars

Maxillary Third Molar

Label and color the maxillary third molar.

Fill in the blanks:

1. The maxillary third molar erupts when you are _____ of age.

2. The maxillary third molar is referred to as the _____ tooth.
Why?

3. Do all humans develop maxillary third molars? _____

4. The occlusal surface of the maxillary third molar is more wrinkled in appearance due to many more _____ _____ grooves.

5. The dentist often times recommends that this tooth be _____.

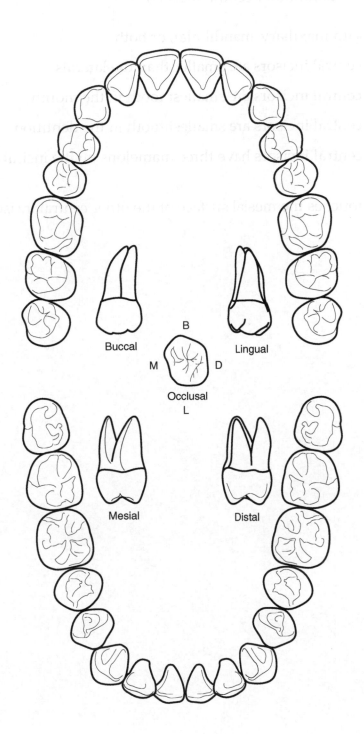

Buccal

Lingual

B

M   D

Occlusal

L

Mesial

Distal

Mandibular Central Incisors

Label and color the mandibular central incisors.

Fill in the blank with maxillary, mandibular, or both.

1. _____ central incisors are smaller than the laterals

2. _____ central incisors are smallest tooth in the mouth

3. _____ central incisors are smallest tooth in the dentition

4. _____ central incisors have three mamelons on the incisal edge
   when erupts

5. _____ touches the mesial surface of the other central incisor

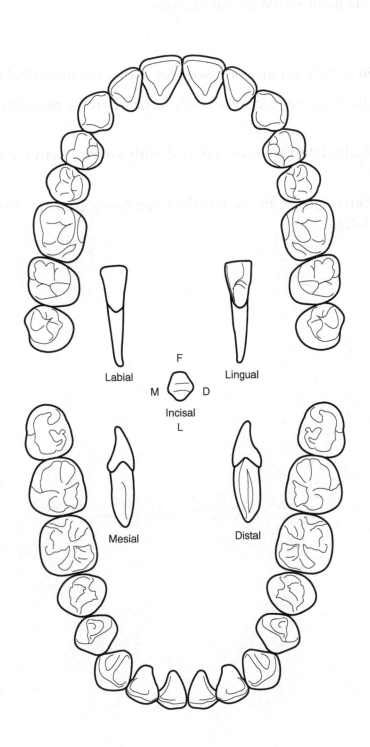

Labial

Lingual

F

M D

Incisal

L

Mesial

Distal

Mandibular Lateral Incisors

Label and color the mandibular lateral incisors.

True or false:

1. _____ mandibular lateral incisor resembles that of the mandibular central incisor.

2. _____ mandibular lateral incisor slightly larger than the mandibular central incisor.

3. _____ mandibular lateral incisor root is slightly shorter than the mandibular central incisor.

4. _____ mandibular lateral incisor has the same developmental abnormalities as the maxillary lateral.

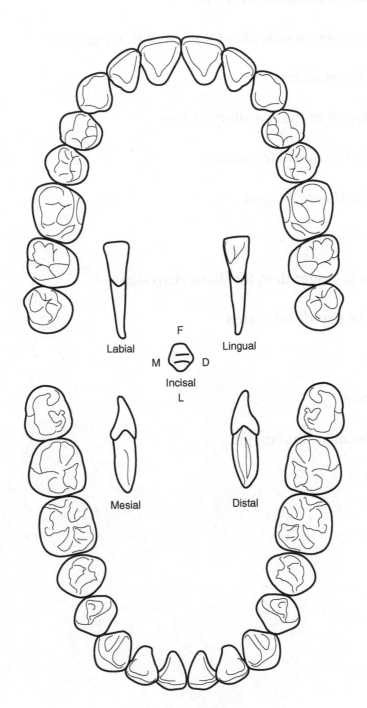

Mandibular lateral incisors

Mandibular Cuspids

Label and color the mandibular cuspids.

Circle all of the true statements about the mandibular cuspids:

third tooth from the midline

not as well developed as the maxillary canine

root is longer than the maxillary canine

not as sharp on the tip of the apex

designed to chew food

mesial cusp slope is longer than the distal cusp slope

longest tooth in the mandibular arch

bifurcated

one canal in the root

cornerstone for the mandibular arch

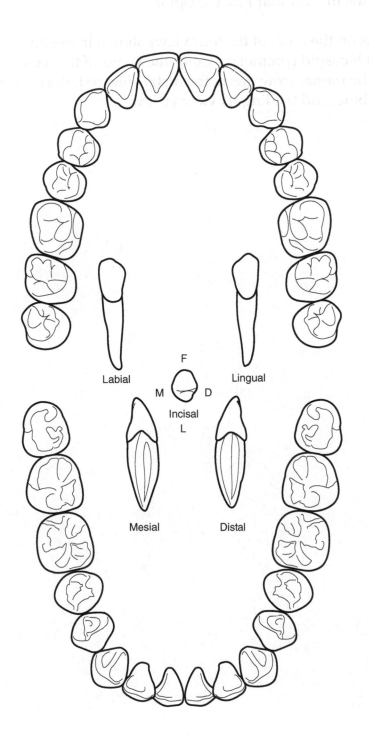

Labial

Lingual

F

M   D

Incisal

L

Mesial

Distal

Mandibular First Bicuspids (Premolars)

Label and color the mandibular first bicuspids.

Draw the crowns on the roots of the four views shown in the line drawing of the mandibular first bicuspid (premolar). Color the views of the teeth shown from five surfaces. Color the mesial view green, the distal view red, the occlusal view orange, the buccal view blue, and the lingual view yellow.

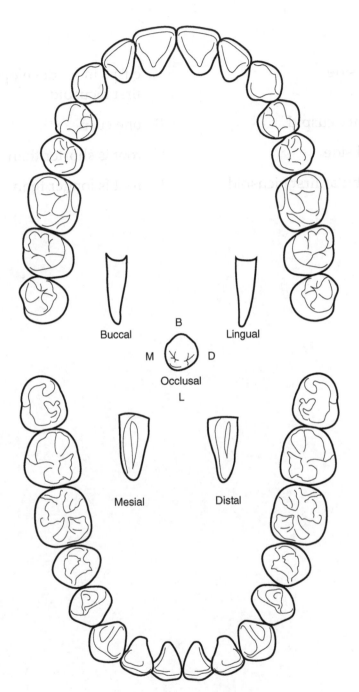

B

Buccal   Lingual

M   D

Occlusal

L

Mesial   Distal

Mandibular first premolars

Mandibular Second Bicuspids (Premolars)

Label and color the mandibular second bicuspids.

Mix and match:

1. _____ buccal side

2. _____ maxillary cuspid

3. _____ lingual side

4. _____ mandibular first bicuspid

A. cusps more developed than first bicuspid

B. one cusp

C. root is shorter than

D. root is longer than

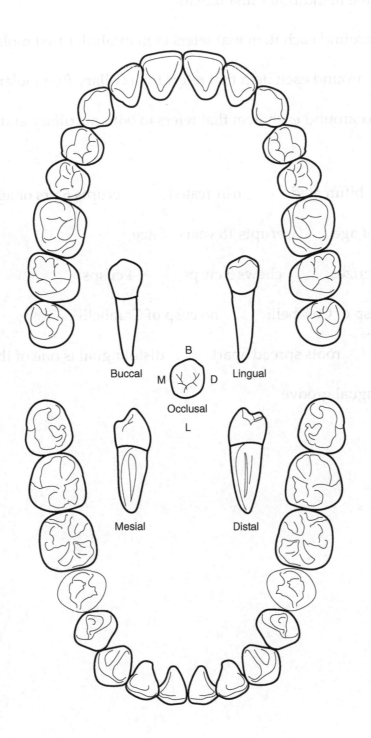

Buccal

B

M   D

Occlusal

L

Lingual

Mesial

Distal

Mandibular First Molar

Label and color the mandibular first molars.

Color a red box around each item that refers to mandibular first molar.

Color a blue box around each item that refers to maxillary first molar.

Color a green box around each item that refers to both maxillary and mandibular first molars.

single root   bifurcated   trifurcated   erupts 6 yrs of age

erupts 12 years of age   erupts 18 years of age

tears   pulverizes   chews 3 cusps   4 cusps

5 cusps   cusp of Carabelli   no cusp of Carabelli

roots together   roots spread apart   distolingual is one of the largest cusps

buccal groove lingual groove

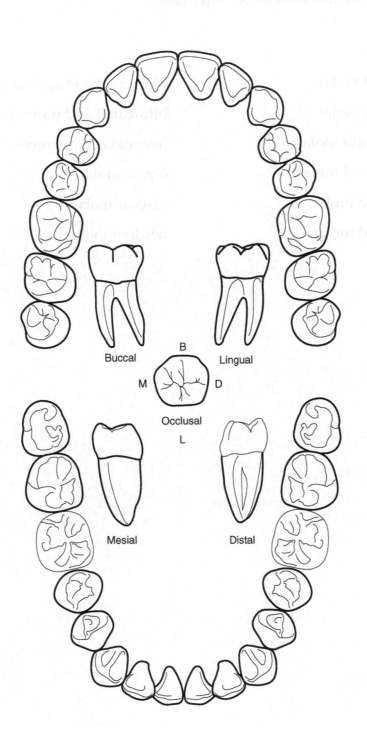

Buccal

Lingual

B

M   D

Occlusal

L

Mesial   Distal

Mandibular Second Molar

Label and color the mandibular second molars.

Mix and match:

mandibular first molar	bifurcated and spread apart the most
mandibular first molar	bifurcated and roots closer together
mandibular second molar	may have many roots
mandibular second molar	6-year molar
mandibular third molar	12-year molar
mandibular third molar	wisdom tooth

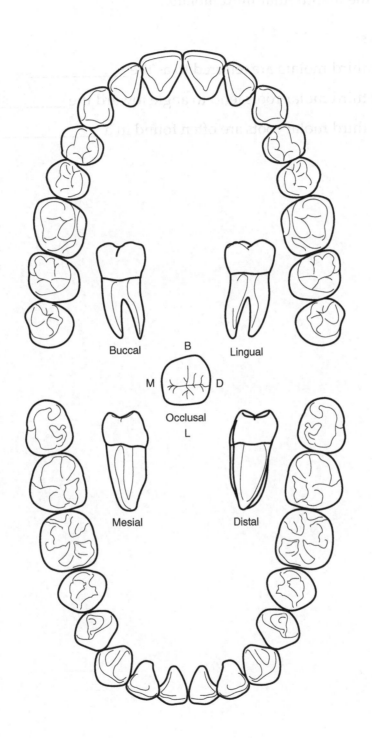

Buccal

B

Lingual

M D

Occlusal

L

Mesial

Distal

Mandibular Third Molar

Label and color the mandibular third molars.

Fill in the blanks:

The mandibular third molars are referred to as the _____.

The mandibular third molar roots tend to angle toward the _____.

The mandibular third molar roots are often found in a _____ position.

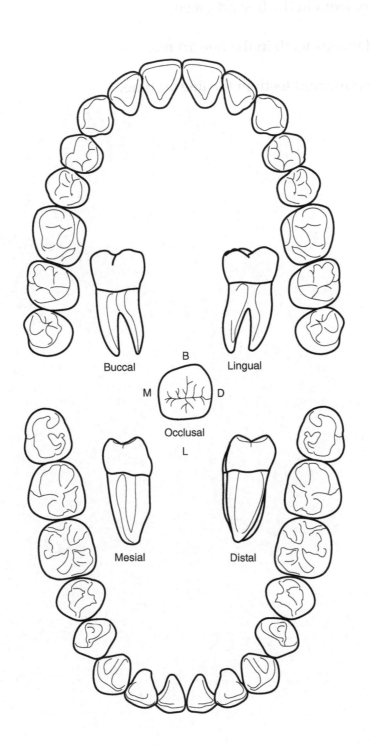

Buccal

B

Lingual

M ⌒ D

Occlusal

L

Mesial

Distal

Mixed Dentition of a Seven- or Eight-Year-Old

Color the primary teeth in the line art green.

Color the succedaneous teeth in the line art red.

Color the other permanent teeth in the line art blue.

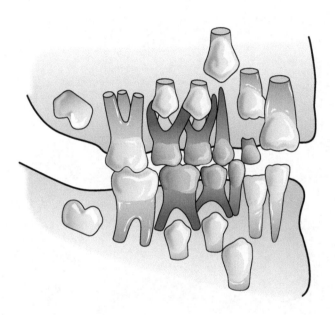

Contact and Embrasure

Label and color the occlusal embrasure with red.

Label and color the lingual embrasure with blue.

Label and color the facial embrasure with green.

Label and color the gingival embrasure with orange.

Make a black X on the contact point on each of the line art.

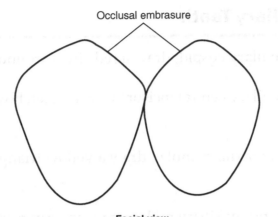

Occlusal embrasure

Facial view

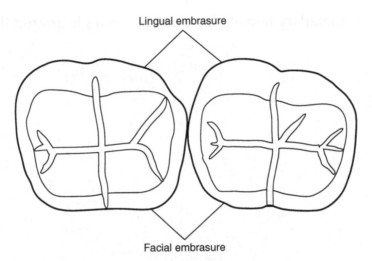

Lingual embrasure

Facial embrasure

Occlusal view

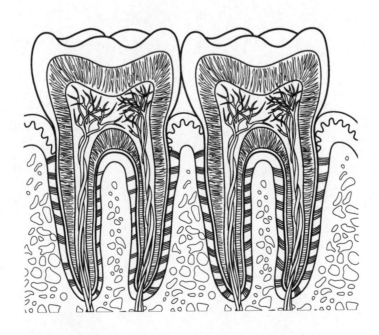

Deciduous Maxillary Teeth

Find the deciduous maxillary cuspid, draw a red circle around it, and color it red.

Find the deciduous maxillary central incisor, draw a green box around it, and color it green.

Find the deciduous first maxillary molar, draw a yellow triangle around it, and color it yellow.

Find the deciduous second maxillary molar, draw an orange star over it, and color it orange.

Find the deciduous maxillary lateral, draw a blue rectangle around it, and color it blue.

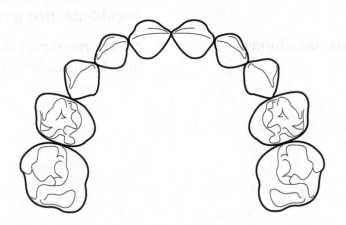

Deciduous Mandibular Teeth

Label and color each of the mandibular deciduous teeth.

Mix and match:

1. _____ mandibular deciduous central incisor

2. _____ mandibular deciduous lateral incisor

3. _____ mandibular deciduous cuspid

4. _____ mandibular deciduous first molar

5. _____ mandibular deciduous second molar

A. resembles no other permanent or deciduous tooth

B. resembles the mandibular deciduous central incisor except that it is slightly longer and wider

C. much more delicate in form than the maxillary deciduous tooth

D. closely resembles the permanent mandibular first molar but is smaller

E. closely resembles the permanent mandibular lateral incisor

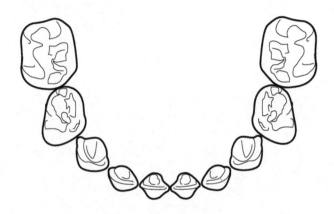

Identification of Teeth

Label each tooth shown.

Identify the maxillary first molar and color it purple.

Identify the mandibular first molar and color it red.

Identify the maxillary cuspid and color it blue.

Identify the mandibular central incisor and color it purple.

Identify the maxillary first bicuspid and color it yellow.

Maxillary

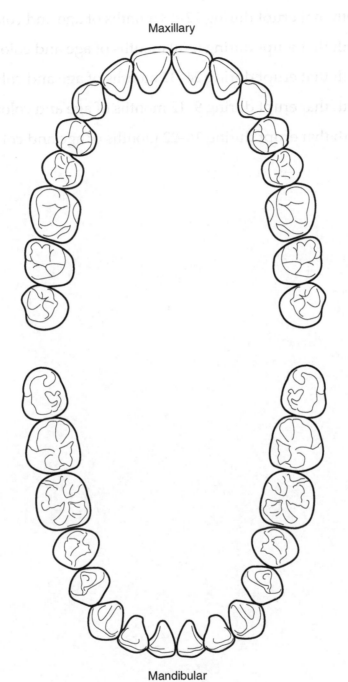

Mandibular

Permanent dentition

Eruption Dates for Primary Teeth

1. Define eruption of teeth.

2. Identify the teeth that erupt during 12–18 months of age and color them blue.

3. Identify the teeth that erupt during 6–10 months of age and color them yellow.

4. Identify the teeth that erupt during 24–32 months of age and color them green.

5. Identify the teeth that erupt during 9–12 months of age and color them red.

6. Identify the teeth that erupt during 16–22 months of age and color them pink.

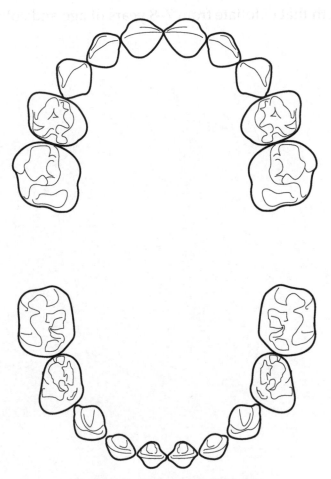

Maxillary deciduous central incisors

Exfoliation Dates for Primary Teeth

1. Define exfoliation of teeth.

2. Identify the teeth that exfoliate from 6–7 years of age and color them pink.

3. Identify the teeth that exfoliate from 10–12 years of age and color them green. (Remember, that includes six teeth.)

4. Identify the teeth that exfoliate from 9–11 years of age and color them red.

5. Identify the teeth that exfoliate from 7–8 years of age and color them blue.

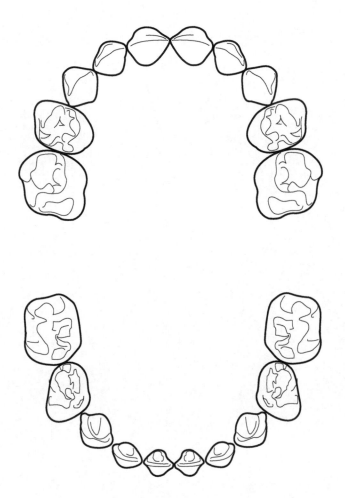

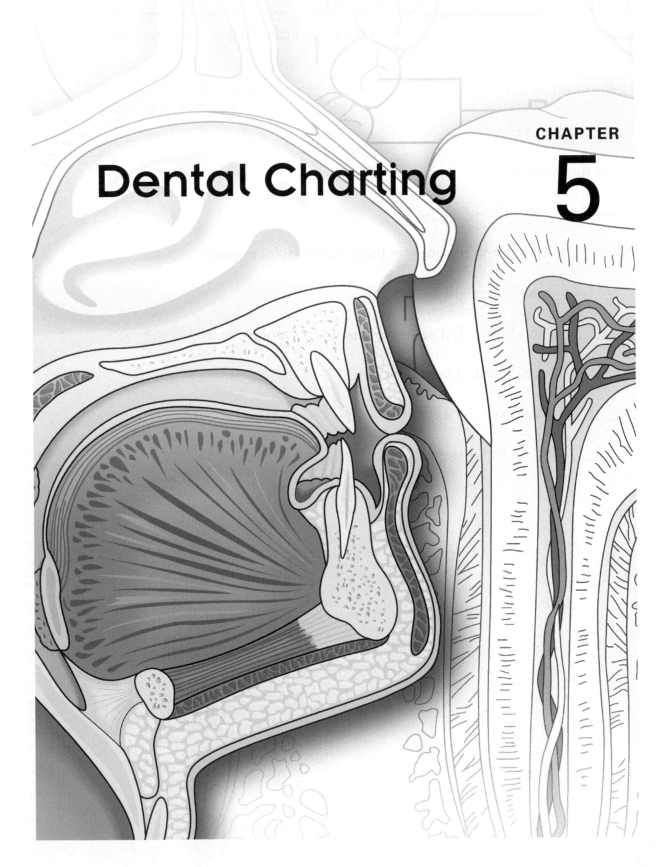

Dental Charting

Universal Numbering System

Number each tooth in the permanent dentition according to the universal numbering system.

Color tooth #3 red.

Color tooth #14 blue.

Color tooth #19 green.

Color tooth #30 yellow.

Fill in the correct tooth number for the permanent teeth listed.

_____ maxillary right first molar

_____ mandibular left second bicuspid (premolar)

_____ maxillary left lateral incisor

_____ maxillary right cuspid

_____ mandibular right third molar

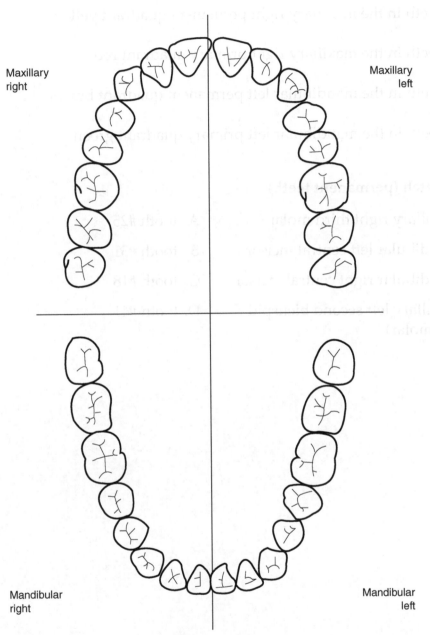

Maxillary right

Maxillary left

Mandibular right

Mandibular left

Permanent teeth

International Standards Organization Numbering System

Number each quadrant and tooth in both the permanent dentition and the primary dentition.

Color the teeth in the maxillary right permanent quadrant yellow.

Color the teeth in the maxillary right primary quadrant red.

Color the teeth in the mandibular left permanent quadrant blue.

Color the teeth in the mandibular left primary quadrant green.

Mix and match (permanent teeth):

_____ maxillary right third molar   A. tooth #25

_____ mandibular left central incisor   B. tooth #31

_____ mandibular right central incisor   C. tooth #18

_____ maxillary left second bicuspid   D. tooth #41
(premolar)

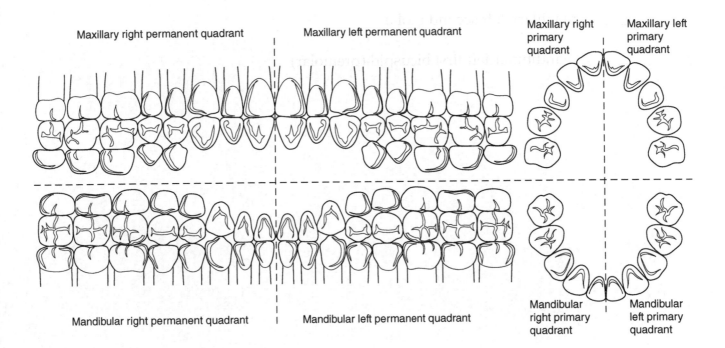

Maxillary right permanent quadrant

Maxillary left permanent quadrant

Maxillary right primary quadrant

Maxillary left primary quadrant

Mandibular right permanent quadrant

Mandibular left permanent quadrant

Mandibular right primary quadrant

Mandibular left primary quadrant

Palmer Numbering System

Label and color each tooth in the permanent and primary dentition the same in each quadrant of the Palmer numbering system. Example: color all lateral incisors green.

Place the correct symbol next to the permanent tooth listed:

_____ maxillary right cuspid

_____ mandibular right first molar

_____ maxillary left lateral incisor

_____ maxillary left second molar

_____ mandibular left first bicuspid (premolar)

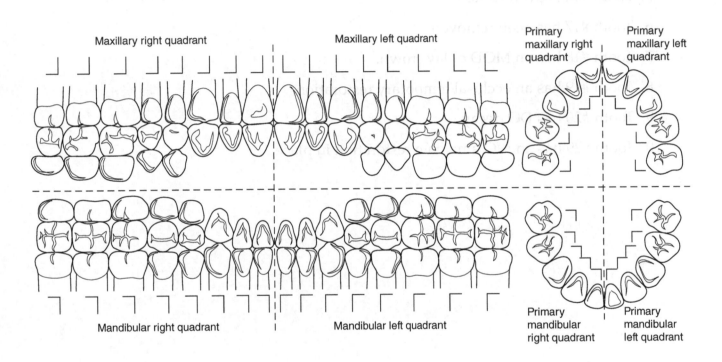

Maxillary right quadrant

Maxillary left quadrant

Primary maxillary right quadrant

Primary maxillary left quadrant

Mandibular right quadrant

Mandibular left quadrant

Primary mandibular right quadrant

Primary mandibular left quadrant

Charting Example #1

Use the charting color indication and symbols on the Universal numbering system for the following:

1. Tooth #3 has a Class II MOD amalgam restoration present.

2. Tooth #6 has a Class III Mesial composite restoration in place with recurrent decay.

3. Tooth #8 has had a root canal treatment, apicoectomy, and a silver retrofilling.

4. Tooth #13 has an abcess and needs a root canal.

5. Tooth #16 is overerupted.

6. Tooth #17 has been removed.

7. Tooth #18 has an MOD onlay crown.

8. Tooth #19 has an occlusal temporary restoration.

9. Tooth #20 has DO decay.

10. Tooth #29 has an MO amalgam restoration in place.

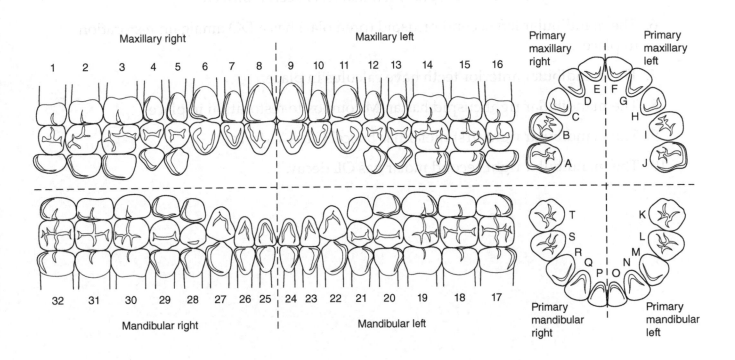

Maxillary right

Maxillary left

Primary maxillary right

Primary maxillary left

1 2 3 4 5 6 7 8 9 10 11 12 13 14 15 16

E F
D G
C H
B I
A J

32 31 30 29 28 27 26 25 24 23 22 21 20 19 18 17

Mandibular right

Mandibular left

T K
S L
R M
Q N
P O

Primary mandibular right

Primary mandibular left

Charting Example #2

Use the charting color indication and symbols on the Universal numbering system for the following:

1. The maxillary right second molar has MO decay.

2. The maxillary right first molar needs a full gold crown.

3. The maxillary right cuspid has MI decay.

4. The maxillary right lateral is missing and the primary tooth is remaining in place.

5. The maxillary left first bicuspid (premolar) has been removed.

6. The mandibular left second bicuspid (premolar) has a DO amalgam restoration in place.

7. The mandibular anterior teeth have calculus in place.

8. The mandibular right cuspid has an M composite restoration in place.

9. The mandibular right first molar has buccal Class V decay.

10. The mandibular right second molar has OL decay.

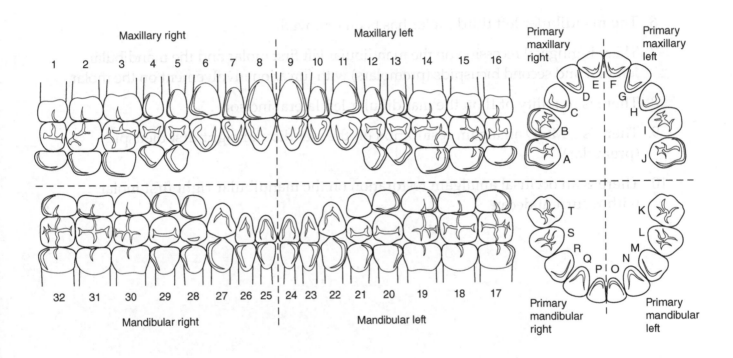

Maxillary right   Maxillary left

1   2   3   4   5   6   7   8 | 9   10   11   12   13   14   15   16

32   31   30   29   28   27   26   25 | 24   23   22   21   20   19   18   17

Mandibular right   Mandibular left

Primary maxillary right

Primary maxillary left

Primary mandibular right

Primary mandibular left

Charting Example #3

Use the charting color indication and symbols on the Universal numbering system for the following:

1. The maxillary right first molar has a stainless steel crown in place.

2. The maxillary right second bicuspid is rotated.

3. The maxillary right cuspid has a distal composite in place with recurrent decay.

4. The maxillary right lateral has an implant in place with a full porcelain crown.

5. There is a diastema between the maxillary right central incisor and the maxillary left central incisor.

6. The mandibular left third molar has been removed.

7. There is gingival recession on the mandibular left first molar and the mandibular left first and second bicuspids (premolars) with furcation involvement on the molar.

8. There is mobility of II on the mandibular left lateral incisor.

9. There is a MOD amalgam restoration on the mandibular right first bicuspid (premolar).

10. There is an occlusal amalgam restoration on the mandibular right first molar with recurrent decay.

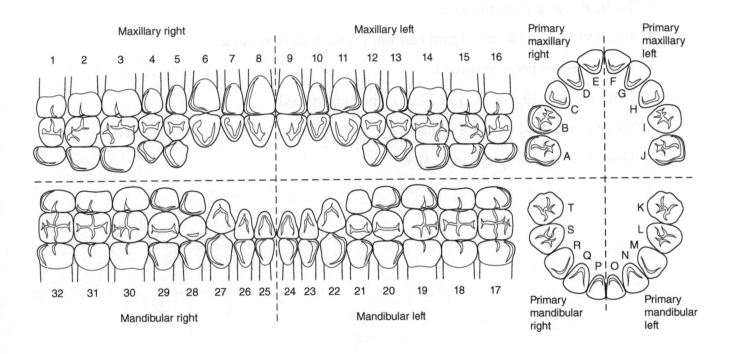

Maxillary right   Maxillary left   Primary maxillary right   Primary maxillary left

1 2 3 4 5 6 7 8 | 9 10 11 12 13 14 15 16

Mandibular right   Mandibular left

32 31 30 29 28 27 26 25 | 24 23 22 21 20 19 18 17

Primary mandibular right   Primary mandibular left

Charting Example #4

Use the charting color indication and symbols on the Universal numbering system for the following:

1. Tooth #1 has been removed.

2. Tooth #2 has MO decay.

3. Teeth #3–5 are a bridge and tooth #4 is missing, tooth #3 is a full gold abutment, tooth #4 is a porcelain with gold abutment, tooth #5 is a porcelain with gold abutment.

4. There is a supernumerary tooth above tooth #8.

5. Tooth #9 has a D composite.

6. Tooth #14 has a DO amalgam restoration with an overhang.

7. Tooth #16 has been removed.

8. Teeth #17, 18, 19, 30, 31, and 32 have been removed.

9. There is a partial denture replacing the mandibular teeth #18, 19, 30, and 31.

10. There is III mobility on tooth #24.

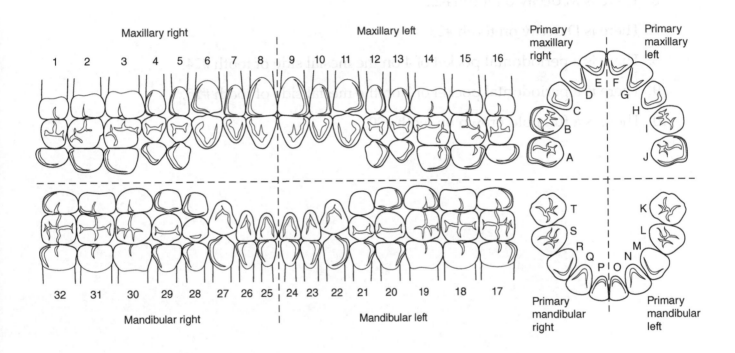

Maxillary right

Maxillary left

Primary maxillary right

Primary maxillary left

1 2 3 4 5 6 7 8 9 10 11 12 13 14 15 16

E F
D G
C H
B I
A J

32 31 30 29 28 27 26 25 24 23 22 21 20 19 18 17

Mandibular right

Mandibular left

T K
S L
R M
Q N
P O

Primary mandibular right

Primary mandibular left

Charting Example #5

Use the charting color indication and symbols on the Universal numbering system for the following:

1. All the maxillary teeth have been removed.

2. There is a full denture in place on the maxillary arch.

3. The mandibular left third molar has been removed.

4. There is a full gold crown on tooth #18.

5. There is an MO amalgam restoration on tooth #19.

6. There is M decay on tooth #22.

7. There is D decay on tooth #23.

8. There is a periodontal pocket of 4 on the mesial side of tooth #24.

9. There is a periodontal pocket of 3 on the mesial side of tooth #25.

10. There is a full gold crown on tooth #30.

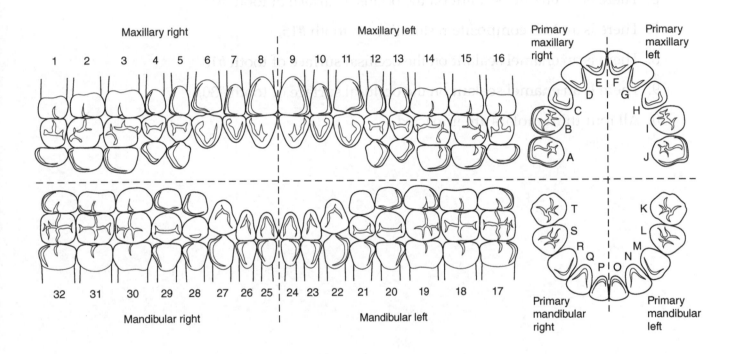

Maxillary right

Maxillary left

Primary maxillary right

Primary maxillary left

1 2 3 4 5 6 7 8 9 10 11 12 13 14 15 16

32 31 30 29 28 27 26 25 24 23 22 21 20 19 18 17

Mandibular right

Mandibular left

Primary mandibular right

Primary mandibular left

Charting Example #6

Use the charting color indication and symbols on the Universal numbering system for the following:

1. There is an MO amalgam on tooth #3.

2. There is a DO amalgam on tooth #4.

3. There is food impaction between teeth #3 and #4.

4. There is a lingual composite, Class 1, on tooth #7.

5. There is decalcification on the facial surface of tooth #9.

6. There is an enamel sealant on the occlusal surface of tooth #14.

7. There is an MO composite restoration on tooth #15.

8. There is an enamel sealant on the occlusal surface of tooth #18.

9. There is an enamel sealant on the occlusal surface of tooth #30.

10. All four third molars are impacted.

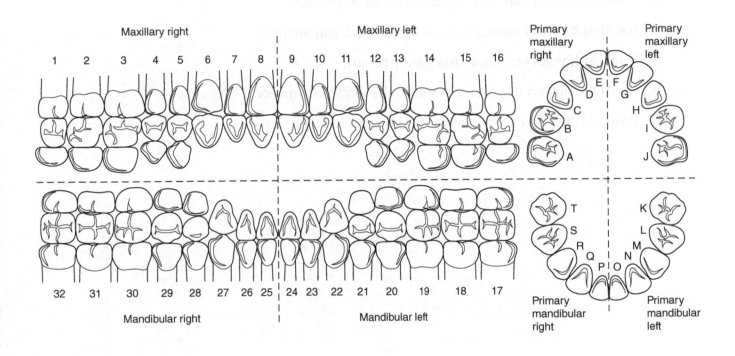

Maxillary right

Maxillary left

Primary maxillary right

Primary maxillary left

1 2 3 4 5 6 7 8 9 10 11 12 13 14 15 16

E F
D G
C H
B I
A J

32 31 30 29 28 27 26 25 24 23 22 21 20 19 18 17

Mandibular right

Mandibular left

Primary mandibular right

Primary mandibular left

T K
S L
R M
Q N
P O

Charting Example #7

Use the charting color indication and symbols on the Universal numbering system for the following:

1. All the primary anterior teeth are missing.

2. The third molars are impacted.

3. The permanent maxillary right second molar has occlusal decay.

4. The permanent bicuspids (premolars) are impacted.

5. Tooth #A has a DO amalgam restoration present.

6. Tooth #B has an MO amalgam restoration present.

7. Tooth #I has an enamel sealant on the occlusal surface.

8. Tooth #J has an occlusal amalgam present.

9. Tooth #K has an enamel sealant on the occlusal surface.

10. Tooth #T has an enamel sealant on the occlusal surface.

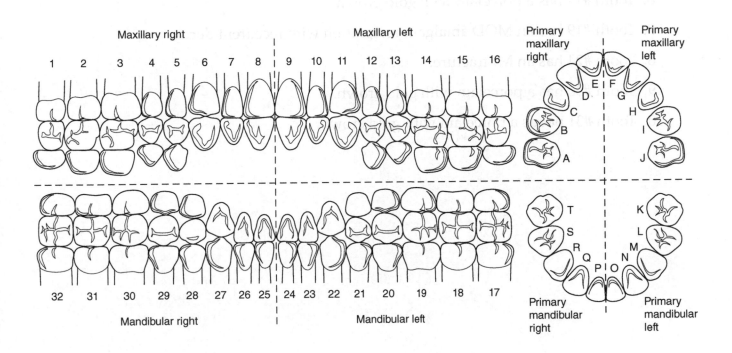

Maxillary right   Maxillary left

1 2 3 4 5 6 7 8 | 9 10 11 12 13 14 15 16

Primary maxillary right   Primary maxillary left

E F
D   G
C   H
B   I
A   J

32 31 30 29 28 27 26 25 | 24 23 22 21 20 19 18 17

Mandibular right   Mandibular left

T   K
S   L
R   M
Q   N
P O

Primary mandibular right   Primary mandibular left

Charting Example #8

Use the charting color indication and symbols on the Universal numbering system for the following:

1. Tooth #3 has an abscess and needs root canal therapy.

2. Tooth #4 has an MO composite restoration in place.

3. Tooth #7 has a lingual decay.

4. Tooth #8 has a porcelain veneer.

5. Tooth #9 has a porcelain veneer.

6. Tooth #14 has a porcelain with gold crown.

7. Tooth #19 has an MOD amalgam restoration with reccurent decay.

8. Tooth #24 has an MI fracture.

9. Tooth #30 has a porcelain with gold crown.

10. Tooth #31 needs a porcelain with gold crown.

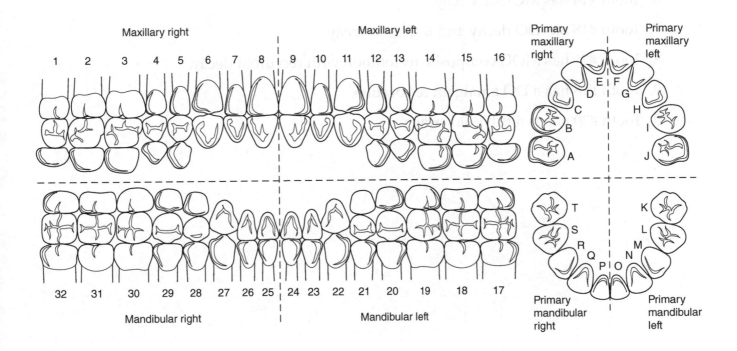

Maxillary right

Maxillary left

1 2 3 4 5 6 7 8 9 10 11 12 13 14 15 16

32 31 30 29 28 27 26 25 24 23 22 21 20 19 18 17

Mandibular right

Mandibular left

Primary maxillary right

Primary maxillary left

E F
D G
C H
B I
A J

T K
S L
R M
Q N
P O

Primary mandibular right

Primary mandibular left

Charting Example #9

Use the charting color indication and symbols on the Universal numbering system for the following:

1. Tooth #1 is impacted.

2. Tooth #2 has an MO decay.

3. Tooth #4 has a DO composite restoration.

4. Tooth #7 has a full porcelain crown.

5. Tooth #8 has a DI fracture.

6. Tooth #14 has MODBL decay.

7. Tooth #18 has DO decay and B class V decay.

8. Tooth #21 has MOD composite restoration with reccurent decay.

9. Tooth #28 has a DO amalgam restoration.

10. Tooth #30 needs a full gold crown.

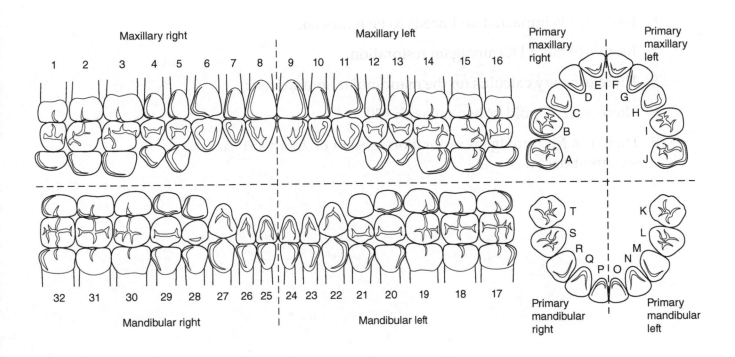

Maxillary right

1 2 3 4 5 6 7 8 9 10 11 12 13 14 15 16

Maxillary left

Primary maxillary right

Primary maxillary left

E F
D G
C H
B I
A J

32 31 30 29 28 27 26 25 24 23 22 21 20 19 18 17

Mandibular right

Mandibular left

Primary mandibular right

Primary mandibular left

T K
S L
R M
Q N
P O

Charting Example #10

Use the charting color indication and symbols on the Universal numbering system for the following:

1. Tooth #1 needs to be removed.

2. Tooth #3 has MODBL composite restoration.

3. There is a bridge between teeth #7–9. Tooth #8 has been removed. The abutments and the pontic are all porcelain with metal.

4. Tooth #12 has an implant in place and a full porcelain with metal crown.

5. Tooth #16 is overerupted and needs to be removed.

6. Tooth #17 is impacted and needs to be removed.

7. Tooth #19 has a DO amalgam restoration.

8. There is heavy calculus on the mandibular anterior teeth.

9. There is a full gold crown on tooth #30.

10. There is a MO amalgam restoration present on tooth #31 that has reccurent decay.

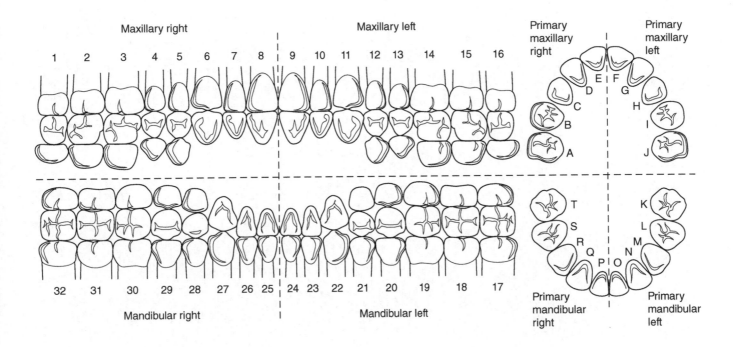

Maxillary right   Maxillary left   Primary maxillary right   Primary maxillary left

1 2 3 4 5 6 7 8 9 10 11 12 13 14 15 16

E F
D G
C H
B I
A J

32 31 30 29 28 27 26 25 24 23 22 21 20 19 18 17

Mandibular right   Mandibular left

T K
S L
R Q P O N M

Primary mandibular right   Primary mandibular left

Introduction to the Dental Office and Basic Chairside Assisting

Small Dental Office Blueprint

1. How many treatment rooms does this office have? _____

Identify and label each of the treatment rooms.

Label the following areas on the diagram: reception area, business area, sterilizing area, lab area, panoramic machine, X-ray processing room, dentist's private office, and staff area.

What small equipment items would be found in the treatment rooms?

_____

Mix and match—identify which room/area the following equipment is found:

1. _____ lab area   A. patient files

2. _____ sterilizing area   B. high-speed dental handpiece

3. _____ treatment room   C. safe light

4. _____ X-ray processing   D. model trimmer
   room

5. _____ business area   E. ultrasonic unit

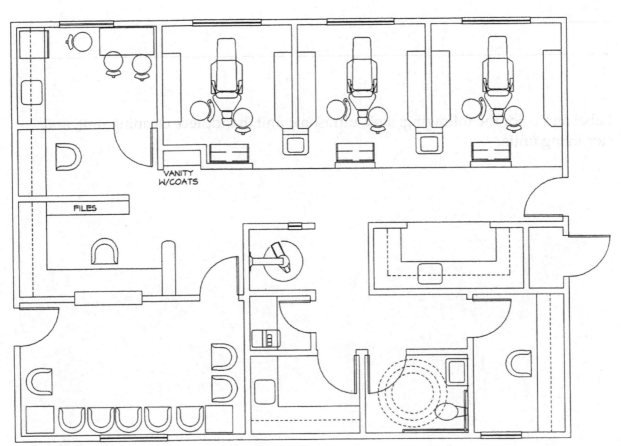

FILES

VANITY
W/COATS

Courtesy of Burkhart Dental Supply

Sterilizing Area

List the items found in the sterilizing area:

_____

_____

_____

_____

_____

Label and color the following: sink, ultrasonic unit, handpiece cleaning unit, and sterilizing units.

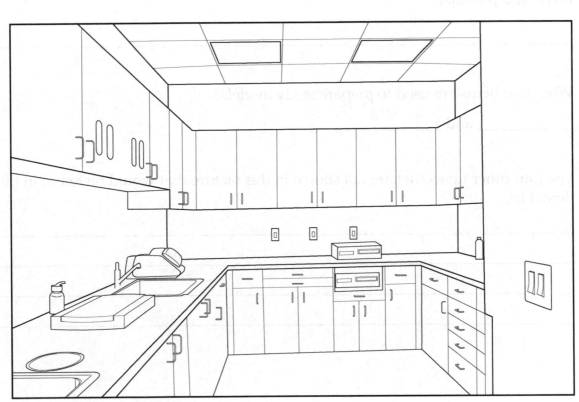

Courtesy of Dr. Jay Enzler

Laboratory Area

Draw an arrow and label the vacuum former.

Draw an arrow and label the dental lathe.

Draw an arrow and label the model trimmer.

Draw an arrow and label the vibrator.

1. Which of the items found in the lab is used to smooth and trim dentures, custom trays, and partials?

   _____

2. What two items are used to prepare study models?

   _____ and _____

3. List four other items that are not shown in this picture that would be found in the dental lab:

   _____

   _____

   _____

   _____

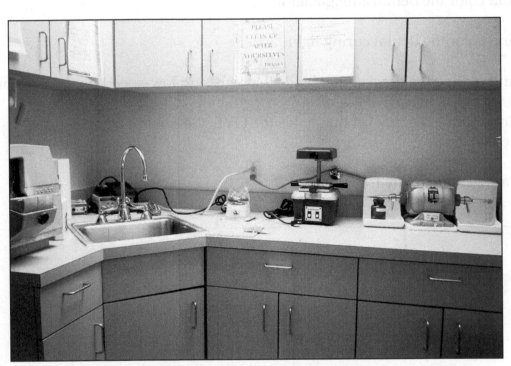

Courtesy of Drs. Rodney Braun and Chris Chaffin

Dental Treatment Room

Label and color the patient chair, the operator's chair, and the assistant's chair.

Label and color the dental light.

Label and color the rheostat.

Label and outline the X-ray view box.

Label and color the dental amalgamator.

Label and color the dental curing light.

Label and outline the bracket that holds the high- and low-speed dental handpieces.

Label and outline the bracket that holds the HVE, the saliva ejector, and the air-water syringe.

Where are the procedure trays stored?

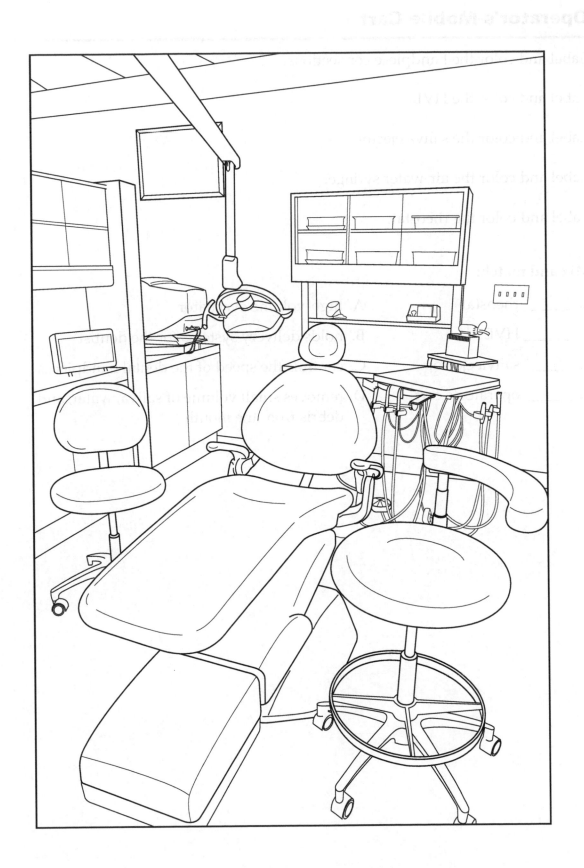

Operator's Mobile Cart

Label and color the handpiece connections.

Label and color the HVE.

Label and color the saliva ejector.

Label and color the air-water syringe.

Label and color the rheostat.

Mix and match:

1. _____ rheostat

2. _____ HVE

3. _____ saliva ejector

4. _____ operator's cart

A. high-volume evacuator

B. holds delivery systems for the dentist

C. controls the speed of the dental handpieces

D. removes small volume of saliva, water, and debris from the mouth

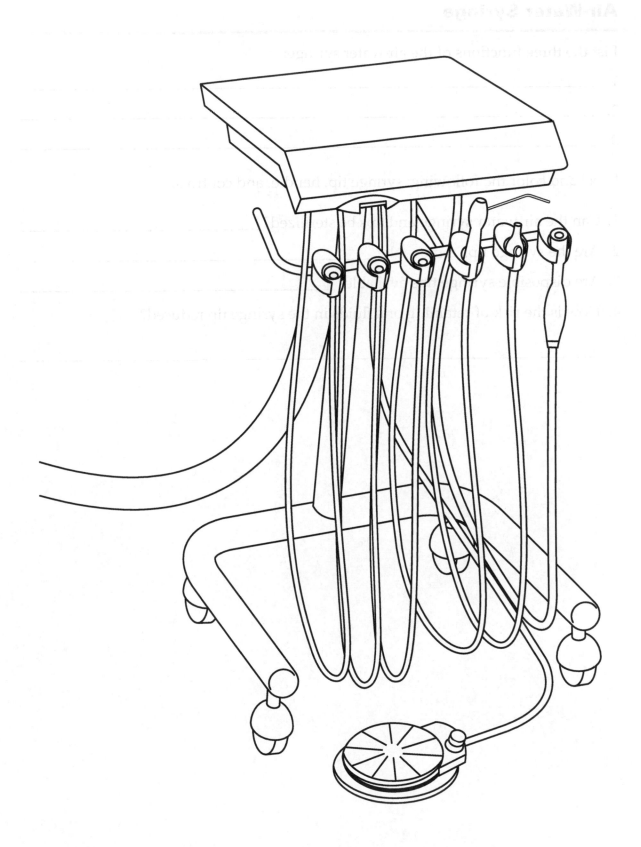

Air-Water Syringe

List the three functions of the air-water syringe:

1. _____

2. _____

3. _____

Label and color the following: syringe tip, handle, and controls.

1. Can the air-water syringe and tips be sterilized? _____

2. Are the syringe tips removable? _____

3. Are disposible syringe tips available? _____

4. How is the risk of retaining oral fluids in the syringe tip reduced?

_____

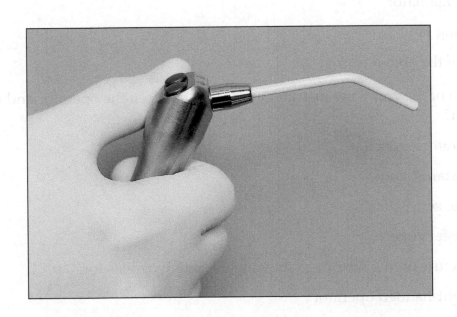

Activity Zones

Label and color the transfer zone.

Label and color the static zone.

Label and color the assistants' zone.

Label and color the operators' zone.

1. Which of the following items would be found in the static zone?

    A. dental instruments

    B. amalgamator

    C. curing light

    D. all of the above

2. In which of the zones are instruments passed between the operator and the assistant?

    A. operators' zone

    B. assistants' zone

    C. static zone

    D. transfer zone

3. Is the picture on the next page showing the activity zones for:

    A. a right-handed operator

    B. a left-handed operator

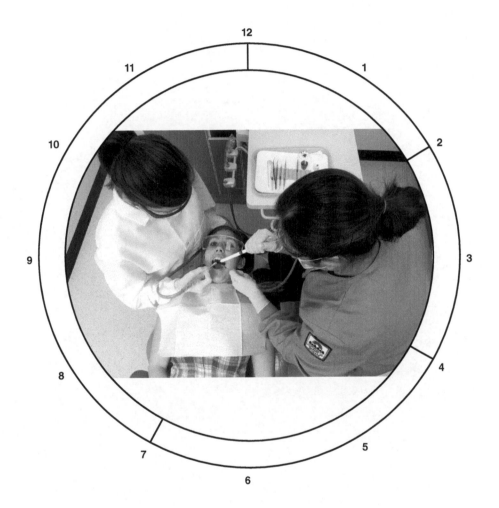

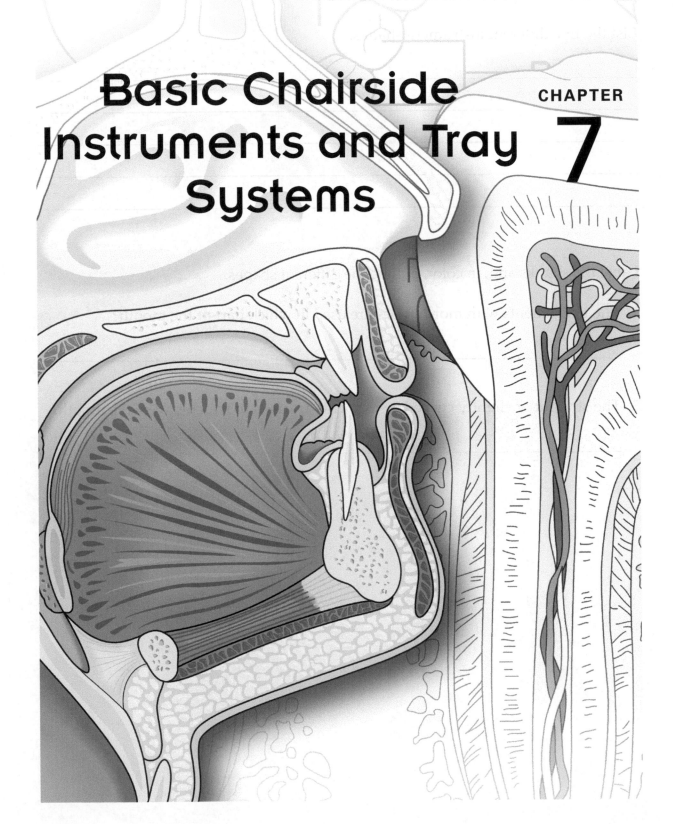

Basic Chairside Instruments and Tray Systems

Parts of an Instrument and Different Shanks

Label and color the parts of a dental instrument.

List the five different instrument shanks:

_____

_____

_____

_____

_____

Label the shanks and, in color, outline the different shapes.

1. The instruments with more angles are used in which part of the mouth?

_____

2. The straight or slightly curved instruments are used in which part of the mouth?

_____

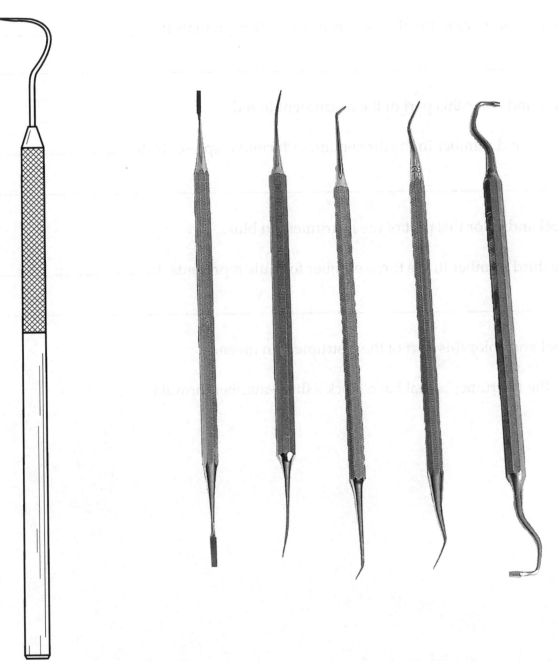

Courtesy of Miltex Instrument Co., Inc., Lake Success, NY

Instruments with Black's Three-Number Formula

Draw a dotted line from the handle extending beyond the working end of the instrument.

The first number in the three-number formula represents the _____

_____.

Label and color this part of the instrument in red.

The second number in the three-number formula represents the _____

_____.

Label and color this part of the instrument in blue.

The third number in the three-number formula represents the _____

_____.

Label and color this part of the instrument in green.

List the instruments that have Black's three-number formula.

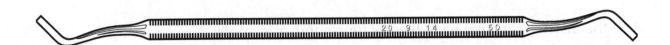

Instruments with Black's Four-Number Formula

Draw a dotted line from the handle extending beyond the working end of the instrument.

The first number in the four-number formula represents the _____.

Label and color this part of the instrument in red.

The second number in the four-number formula represents the _____.

Label and color this part of the instrument in pink.

The third number in the four-number formula represents the _____.

Label and color this part of the instrument in blue.

The fourth number in the four-number formula represents the _____.

Label and color this part of the instrument green.

List the instruments that have Black's four-number formula.

Chisels, Hatchets, and Hoes

Draw a circle around the chisels.

List, label, and outline in color the three chisels.

Label and outline in color the hatchet.

Label and outline in color the hoe.

1. These instruments are called _____.

2. _____ are used in a downward motion to refine the cavity preparation.

3. The _____ chisel is used for Class III and IV cavity preparations.

4. All of these instruments have a _____ edge at the end of the blade.

   A. beveled

   B. bi-beveled

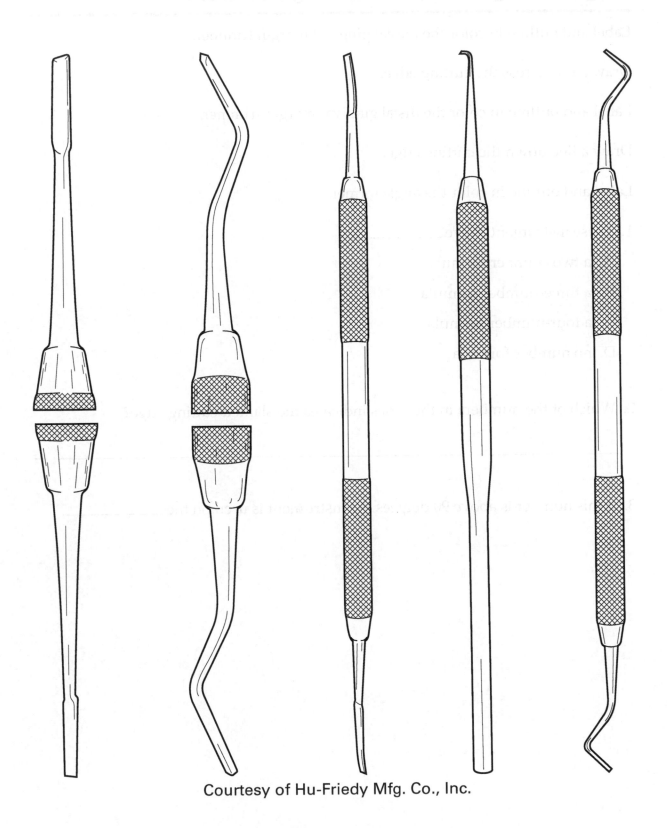

Courtesy of Hu-Friedy Mfg. Co., Inc.

Gingival Margin Trimmers and Angle Formers

Label and outline in color the mesial gingival margin trimmer.

Draw a line across the cutting edge.

Label and outline in color the distal gingival margin trimmer.

Draw a line down the cutting edge.

Label and outline in color the angle former.

1. These instruments have _____.
   A. a two-number formula
   B. a three-number formula
   C. a four-number formula
   D. no number formula

2. Which of the numbers in the series indicates the slanted cutting edge?

   _____

3. If this number is above 90 degrees the instrument is used on the _____.

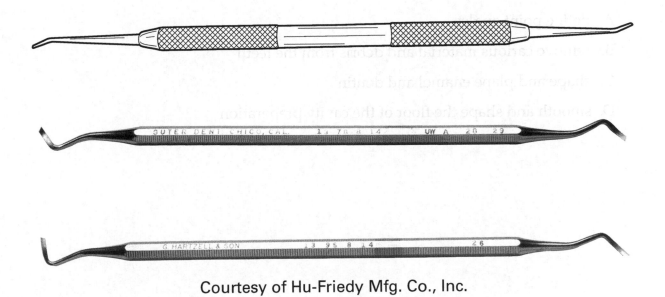

Courtesy of Hu-Friedy Mfg. Co., Inc.

Excavators

1. Another name for excavators is _____.

2. List the two types of excavators:

   _____

   _____

Label and color the working ends of the excavators.

3. Excavators are used to:

   A. define point angles

   B. remove carious material and debris from the teeth

   C. shape and plane enamel and dentin

   D. smooth and shape the floor of the cavity preparation

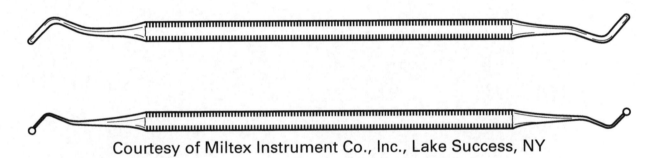

Courtesy of Miltex Instrument Co., Inc., Lake Success, NY

Explorers, Periodontal Probe, and Cotton Pliers

Label and color the double-ended explorer.

Label and color the cotton pliers.

Label and color the instrument that has an explorer on one end and a periodontal probe on the other end.

1. These cotton pliers are _____ pliers.

2. What is the instrument called that has an explorer on one end and a periodontal probe on the other end? _____

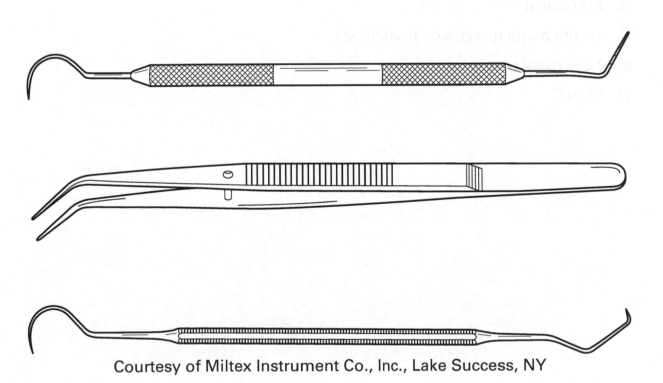

Courtesy of Miltex Instrument Co., Inc., Lake Success, NY

Cement Spatulas and Burnishers

Label and color the cement spatulas.

Label and color the T-ball burnisher.

Label and color the beaver-tail burnisher.

Label and color the football burnisher.

Burnishers are used to:

A. mix cement

B. smooth rough margins on restorations

C. shape metal matrix bands

D. B and C

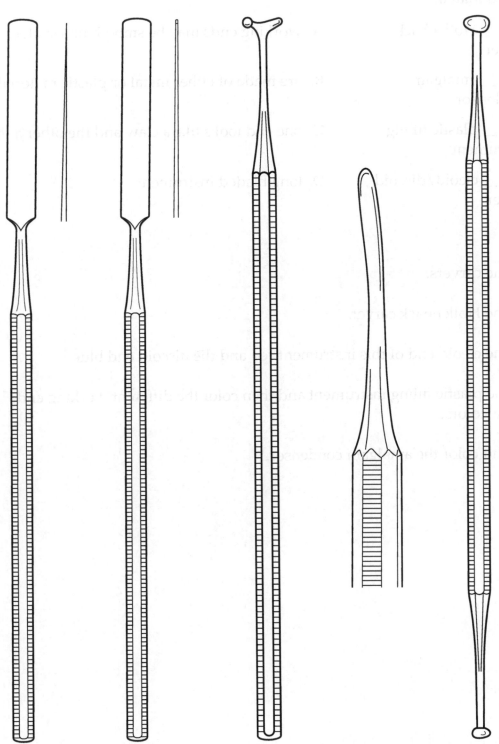

Courtesy of Miltex Instrument Co., Inc., Lake Success, NY

Condensors, Carvers, and Plastic Filling Instruments

Mix and match:

1. _____ Hollenback carver

2. _____ amalgam condensor

3. _____ plastic filling instrument

4. _____ cleoid/discoid carver

A. working ends may be smooth or serrated

B. are made of either metal or plastic materials

C. one end looks like a claw and the other a disc

D. long bladed instrument

Label the carvers.

Color the Hollenback carver.

Color the cleoid end of this instrument red and the discoid end blue.

Label the plastic filling instrument and then color the different working ends different colors.

Label and color the amalgam condensor.

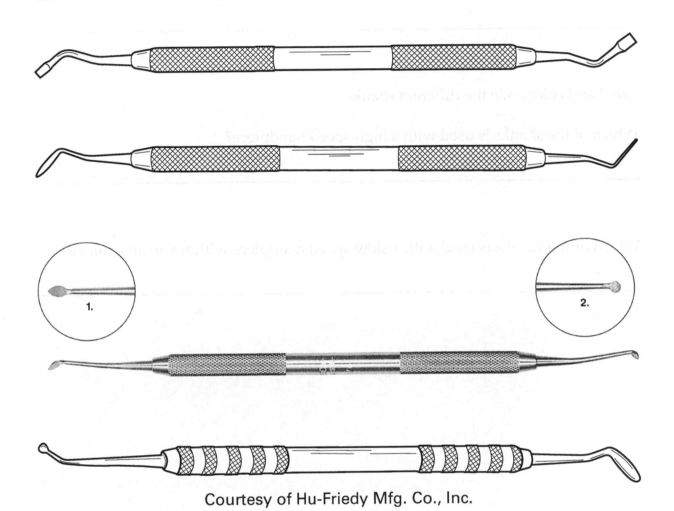

Courtesy of Hu-Friedy Mfg. Co., Inc.

Parts of a Bur and Shanks

Label and color the parts of a bur.

List the three types of shanks on burs:

_____

_____

_____

Label and color code the different shanks.

Which of the shanks is used with a high-speed handpiece?

_____

Which of the shanks is used with a slow-speed handpiece without an attachment?

_____

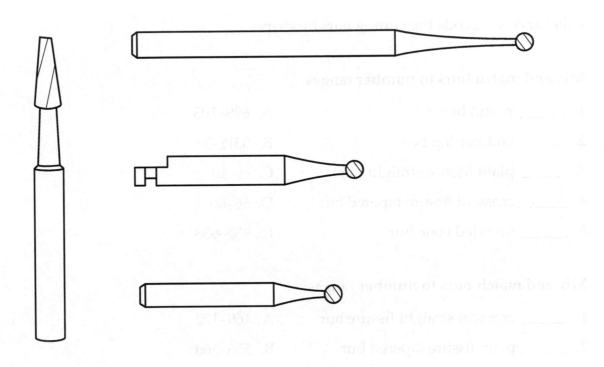

Cutting Bur Shapes and Number Ranges

List the cutting burs:

_____   _____

_____   _____

_____   _____

_____   _____

_____

Label and color code the cutting burs by shape.

Mix and match burs to number ranges:

1. _____ round bur   A. 699–703

2. _____ end-cutting bur   B. 33½–39

3. _____ plain fissure straight bur   C. ¼–10

4. _____ crosscut fissure tapered bur   D. 56–60

5. _____ inverted cone bur   E. 957–958

Mix and match burs to number ranges:

1. _____ crosscut straight fissure bur   A. 169–172

2. _____ plain fissure tapered bur   B. 556–560

3. _____ pear   C. 14

4. _____ wheel   D. 329–332

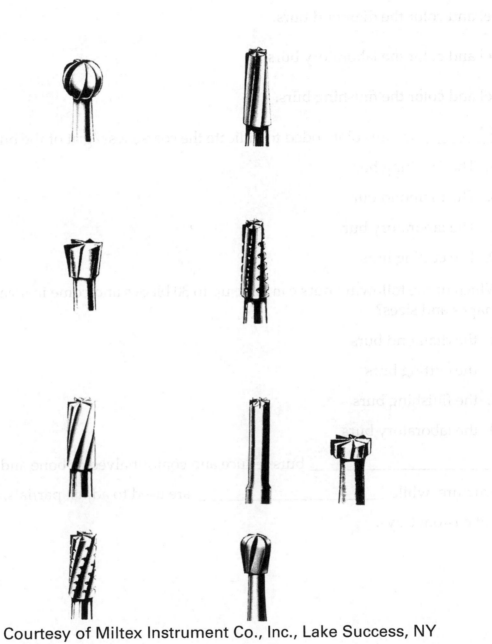

Courtesy of Miltex Instrument Co., Inc., Lake Success, NY

Diamond Burs, Finishing Burs, Surgical Burs, and Laboratory Burs

Label and color the surgical burs.

Label and color the diamond burs.

Label and color the laboratory burs.

Label and color the finishing burs.

1. _____ is/are color coded to indicate the coarseness/grit of the bur.

   A. The finishing bur

   B. The diamond bur

   C. The laboratory bur

   D. The cutting burs

2. Which of the following burs can have up to 30 blades and come in a variety of shapes and sizes?

   A. the diamond burs

   B. the cutting burs

   C. the finishing burs

   D. the laboratory burs

3. _____ burs reduce and contour alveolar bone and tooth structure, while _____ are used to adjust partials, dentures, and custom trays.

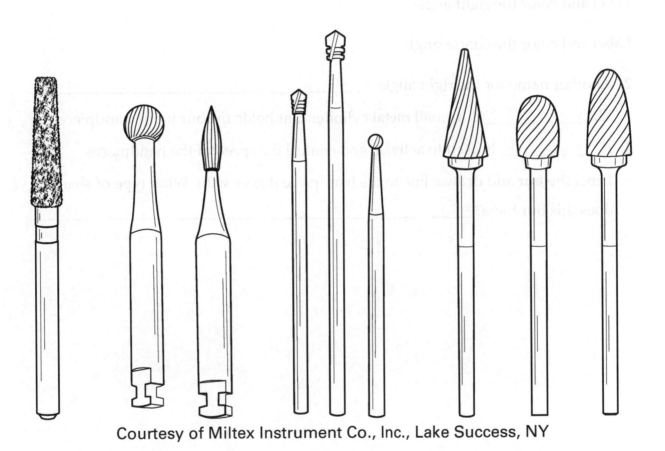

Courtesy of Miltex Instrument Co., Inc., Lake Success, NY

High- and Low-speed Handpieces and Attachments

Label and color the high-speed handpiece.

Label and color the low-speed straight handpiece.

1. Which handpiece has fiber optics? _____

Label and color the fiber optics.

Label and color the right angle.

Label and color the contra-angle.

2. Another name for the right angle is _____.

3. The _____ is a small metal cylinder that holds the bur in the handpiece.

4. A _____ is used to activate and control the speed of the handpieces.

5. Label the bur and draw a line to the handpiece it goes with. What type of shank

   does this bur have? _____

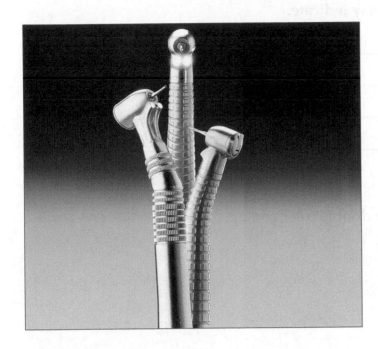

Courtesy of Midwest Dental
Products Corporation,
a division of DENTSPLY
International

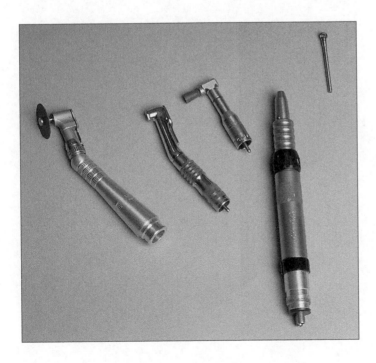

Double Color coding

List what the double color coding may indicate:

_____

_____

_____

_____

Color code the instruments to show double color coding.

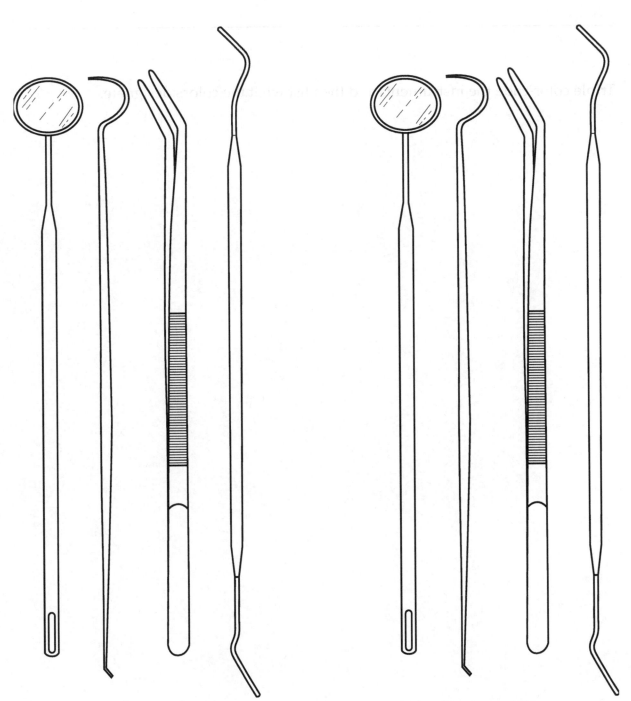

Courtesy of Miltex Instrument Co., Inc., Lake Success, NY

Triple Color coding

When would triple color-coding be necessary?

Triple color-code the instruments and then list what the colors designate.

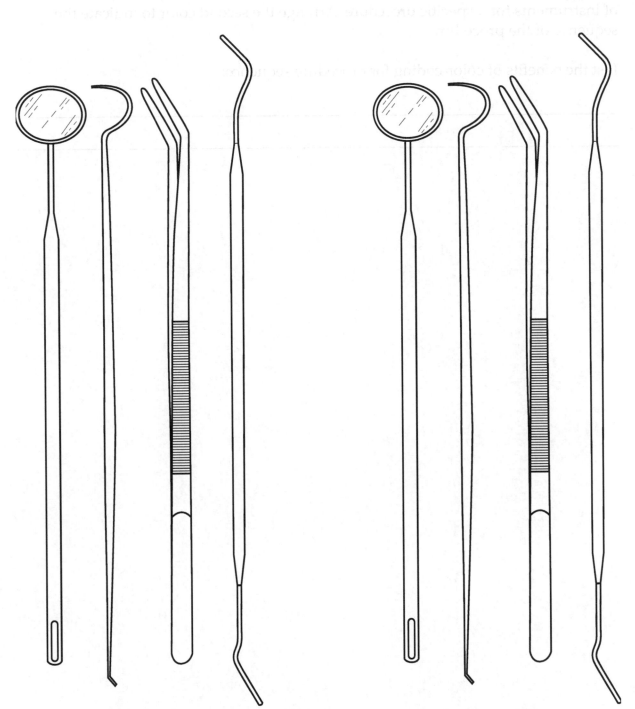

Courtesy of Miltex Instrument Co., Inc., Lake Success, NY

Color-coding for Procedure Sequence

Using double color-coding, color the instruments for the dentist and a second set of instruments for a specific procedure. Arrange the second color to indicate the sequence of the procedure.

List the benefits of color-coding for procedure sequence:

_____

_____

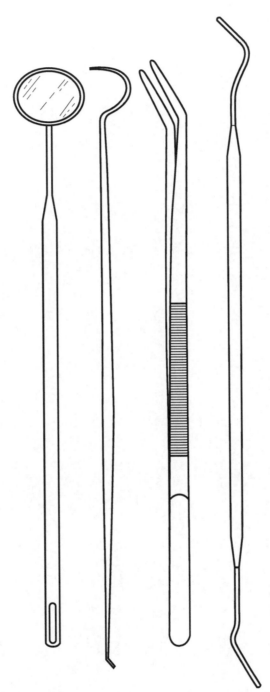

Courtesy of Miltex Instrument Co., Inc., Lake Success, NY

Anesthesia and Sedation

Types of Anesthetic Injections

List the three types of anesthetic injections:

_____

_____

_____

Color the nerve trunk blue.

Color an "X" on the injection site of all three types of anesthetic injections.

Draw a line and label these sites.

Which of the anesthetic injections places the anesthetic near a main nerve trunk?

_____

This anesthetic injection places anesthetic solution into the tissues near the small terminal nerve branches. It is the _____.

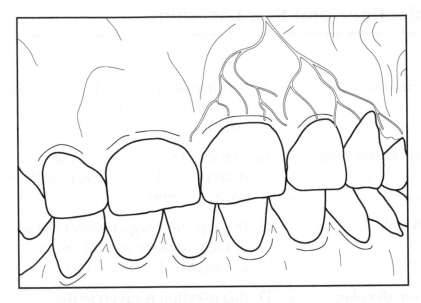

Courtesy of
Dr. Gary Shellerud

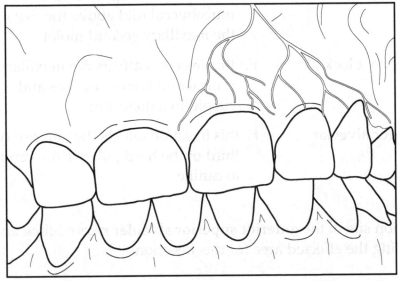

Courtesy of
Dr. Gary Shellerud

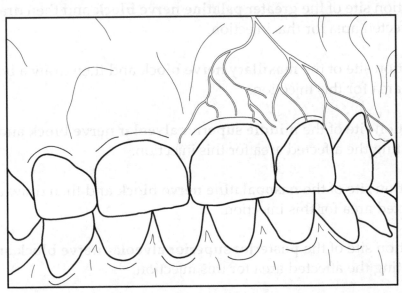

Courtesy of
Dr. Gary Shellerud

Maxillary Arch Injections and Site Locations

Mix and match:

1. _____ anterior superior alveolar nerve block

    A. this injection affects the hard palate and soft tissues covering the hard palate

2. _____ greater palatine nerve block

    B. this injection is given in the muccobuccal fold at the maxillary second premolar

3. _____ maxillary nerve block

    C. this injection is given near the apex of the maxillary second molar toward the distobuccal root

4. _____ middle superior alveolar nerve block

    D. this injection is given in the mucobuccal fold above the distal of the maxillary second molar

5. _____ nasopalatine nerve block

    E. this injection affects the maxillary central and lateral incisors and cuspid in a quadrant

6. _____ posterior superior alveolar nerve block

    F. this injection affects the anterior one-third of the hard palate from canine to canine

Color an "X" at the injection site of the **anterior superior alveolar nerve block** and then draw a box designating the affected area for this injection.

Color an "X" at the injection site of the **greater palatine nerve block** and then draw a box designating the affected area for this injection.

Color an "X" at the injection site of the **maxillary nerve block** and then draw a box designating the affected area for this injection.

Color an "X" at the injection site of the **middle superior alveolar nerve block** and then draw a box designating the affected area for this injection.

Color an "X" at the injection site of the **nasopalatine nerve block** and then draw a box designating the affected area for this injection.

Color an "X" at the injection site of the **posterior superior alveolar nerve block** and then draw a box designating the affected area for this injection.

Maxillary arch

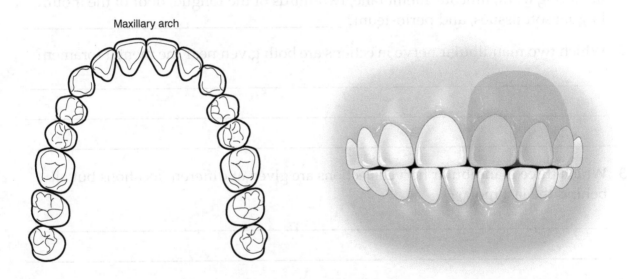

Mandibular Arch Injections and Site Locations

List the mandibular arch injection sites:

_____

_____

_____

_____

_____

1. Which of the mandibular nerve injections affects a mandibular quadrant including teeth, mucous membrane, two-thirds of the tongue, floor of the mouth, lingual soft tissues, and periosteum? _____

2. Which two mandibular nerve injections are both given near the mental foramen?

_____

_____

_____

3. Which three mandibular nerve injections are given at different locations but all behind the last molar?

_____

_____

_____

Color an "X" at the injection site of the **buccal nerve block** and then draw a box designating the affected area for this injection.

Color an "X" at the injection site of the **incisive nerve block** and then draw a box designating the affected area for this injection.

Color an "X" at the injection site of the **inferior alveolar nerve block** and then draw a box designating the affected area for this injection.

Color an "X" at the injection site of the **lingual nerve block** and then draw a box designating the affected area for this injection.

Color an "X" at the injection site of the **mental nerve block** and then draw a box designating the affected area for this injection.

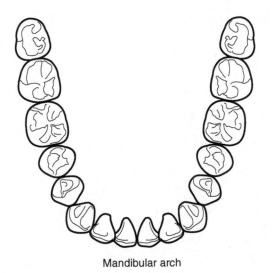

Mandibular arch

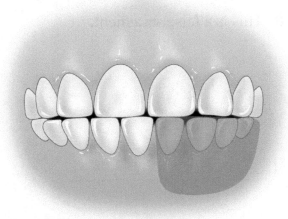

Aspirating Syringe

Label and color the parts of the aspirating syringe:

- needle end
- piston with harpoon
- barrel
- finger grip
- thumb ring

What is another name for the piston rod? _____

All syringes have a harpoon to engage the rubber end of the cartridge.

    A. This is a true statement.

    B. This is a false statement.

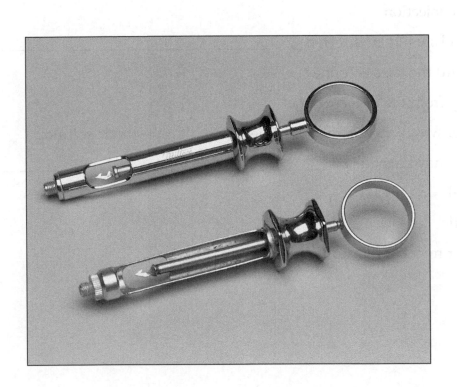

Needle Parts

Label the short needle package and color it blue.

Label the long needle package and color it yellow.

Label and color the following on both the long and short needle: bevel, hub, shank, and syringe end.

1. The long needle is usually used for a(n):

   A. infiltration injection

   B. block injection

2. The bevel should be directed _____.

   A. toward the tissues/bone

   B. away from the tissues/bone

   C. either way; will not affect the injection of the anesthetic solution

3. The hub may be made of _____.

   A. metal

   B. plastic

   C. either metal or plastic

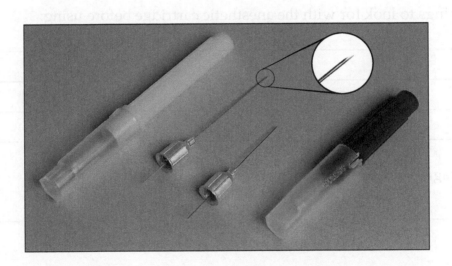

Parts of an Anesthetic Cartridge

List the parts of an anesthetic cartridge:

_____

_____

_____

_____

_____

Label and color the parts of an anesthetic cartridge.

List four things to look for with the anesthetic cartridge before using:

1. _____

2. _____

3. _____

4. _____

The diaphragm is located on which end of the cartridge?

_____

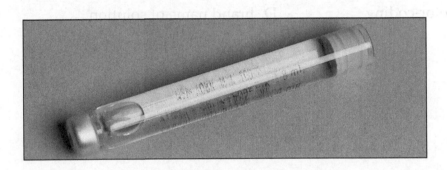

Information on the Anesthetic Cartridge

Label and color the following parts of the anesthetic cartridge: aluminum cap, neck/hub, glass cylinder, rubber diaphragm and rubber stopper

Outline the glass cylinder of the anesthetic cartridge.

List the information found on the anesthetic cartridge:

_____

Mix and match:

1. _____ Mylar plastic label   A. ratio of vasoconstrictor to solution

2. _____ 1:100,000   B. ADA system to identify anesthetics

3. _____ Lidocaine   C. thin plastic cover on all glass cartridges

4. _____ color-coding   D. brand name of solution

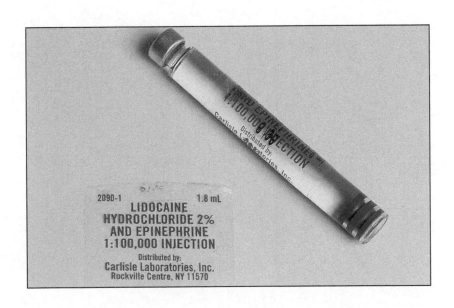

2090-1   1.8 mL
**LIDOCAINE
HYDROCHLORIDE 2%
AND EPINEPHRINE
1:100,000 INJECTION**
Distributed by:
Carlisle Laboratories, Inc.
Rockville Centre, NY 11570

Equipment and Supplies Needed to Prepare an Anesthetic Syringe

Label and outline the anesthetic syringe.

Label the long and short needle, then color the short anesthetic needle blue and the long anesthetic needle yellow.

Draw an arrow to and label the anesthetic cartridges.

Label and color the materials needed to place topical anesthetic.

Draw an arrow to and label the needle holder used for recapping.

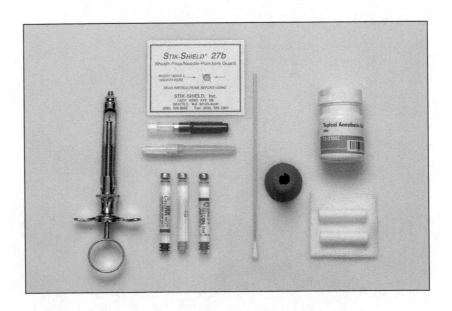

Dental X-ray Film and Holding Devices

Electromagnetic Energy Spectrum and Applications

Color the area where electricity falls on the meter/angstrom scale in red.

Color the area where a television radio and radar would fall on the meter/angstrom scale in yellow.

Color the area on the meter/angstrom scale where a microwave would fall in blue.

Color the area where the sun would fall on the meter/angstrom scale in green.

Color the area where X-rays fall on the meter/angstrom scale in orange.

Match the noted illustrations to the correct area.

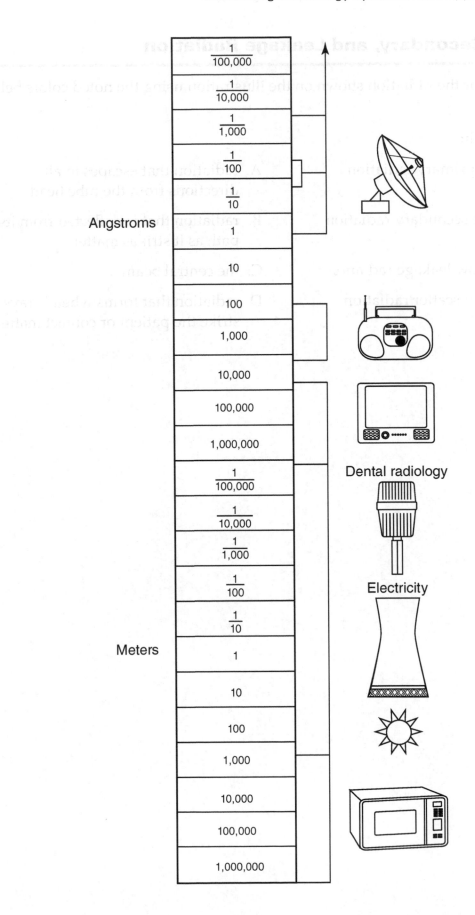

Angstroms

$\frac{1}{100,000}$

$\frac{1}{10,000}$

$\frac{1}{1,000}$

$\frac{1}{100}$

$\frac{1}{10}$

1

10

100

1,000

10,000

100,000

1,000,000

Meters

$\frac{1}{100,000}$

$\frac{1}{10,000}$

$\frac{1}{1,000}$

$\frac{1}{100}$

$\frac{1}{10}$

1

10

100

1,000

10,000

100,000

1,000,000

Dental radiology

Electricity

Primary, Secondary, and Leakage Radiation

Label and color the radiation shown on the illustration using the noted colors below.

Mix and match:

1. _____ red primary radiation

2. _____ blue secondary radiation

3. _____ yellow leakage radiation

4. _____ green scatter radiation

A. radiation that escapes in all directions from the tube head

B. radiation that is deflected from its path as it strikes matter

C. the central beam

D. radiation that forms when X-rays strike the patient or contact matter

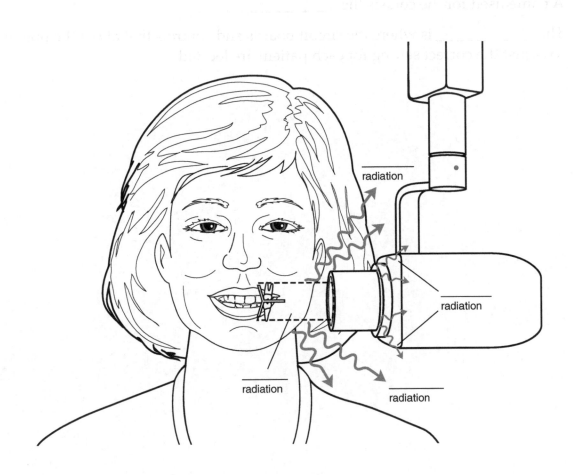

radiation

radiation

radiation

radiation

Parts of Dental Arm Assembly

Identify and color the parts of the dental arm assembly.

1. The _____ allows the operator to freely position the tube head for the various positions required for dental radiography exposures.

2. The _____ is where the X-ray vacuum tube and step down transformers are located.

3. A name used for the cone is the _____.

4. The _____ is where the circuit boards and controls that allow the operator to adjust the correct setting for each patient are located.

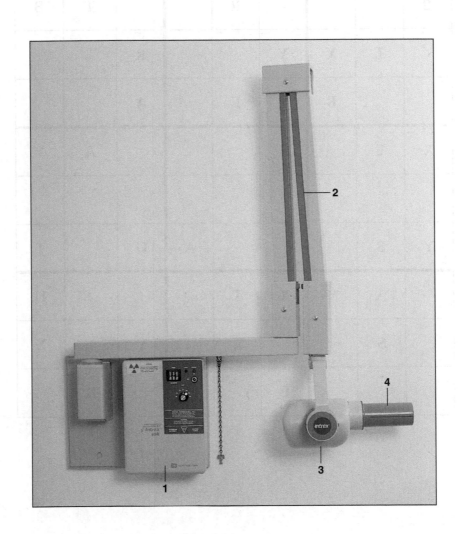

Tube Head, PID, and Vertical Indicator Scale

Label and color the tube head, position indicator device, and the vertical indicator scale.

Using the words "xraytubes," fill out the Sudoku puzzle below.

E				R			T	B
	T	X	Y			R		
		B	T	E		A		
X	E		S				A	Y
Y	B				A	U		T
	A	Y	X	T				U
	S			B		Y		X
			E				B	

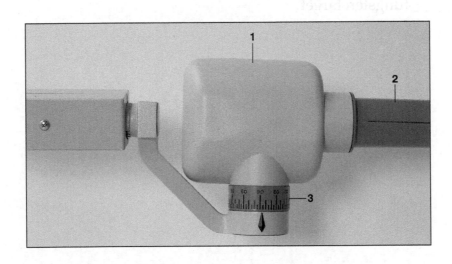

Tube Head and X-ray Tube

Label and color the following devices on the diagram: step up transformer, step down transformer, tungsten filament and focusing cup, tungsten target, anode, cathode, heat radiator, copperstem, lead lining, lead diaphragm (collimator), aluminum filter and metal casing.

Fill in the following with either "cathode" or "anode":

1. _____ negative

2. _____ positive

3. _____ tungsten filament and focusing cup

4. _____ copper stem

5. _____ tungsten target

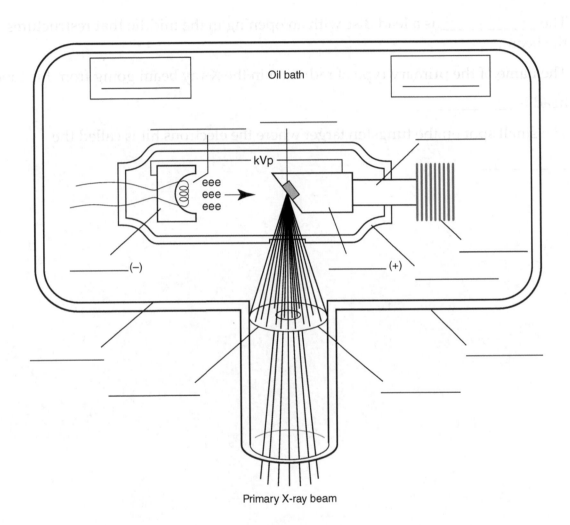

Oil bath

kVp

eee
eee
eee

(−)

(+)

Primary X-ray beam

X-ray Tube

Label and color the following on the X-ray tube: copper stem, aluminum filter, diaphragm, anode, cathode, tungsten filament and focusing cup, tungsten target, glass envelope.

Fill in the blanks:

1. The _____ is a lead disc with an opening in the middle that restructures the beam.

2. The name of the primary type of radiation in the X-ray beam going from the tube head is _____.

3. The small spot on the tungsten target where the electrons hit is called the _____.

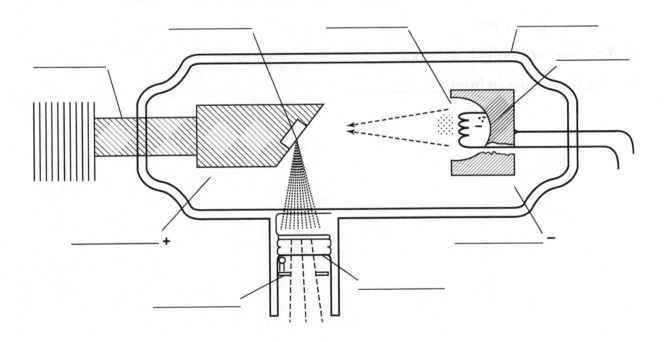

+

−

Composition of Dental X-ray Film

Label and color the composition of a dental X-ray film on the illustration:

emulsion red

transparent base yellow

adhesive layer blue

protective coating layer green

1. A dental X-ray film is composed of a flexible, thin base which is about

   _____ thick.

2. This base normally has a slightly _____ tint to it.

3. This base is made from _____.

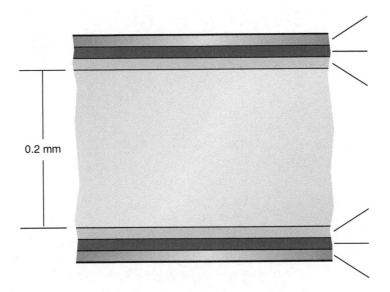

0.2 mm

Sizes of Dental X-ray Film

Label the film sizes and color on the illustration.

Mix and match:

1. _____ adult size

A. No. 0

2. _____ long bite-wing film size

B. No. 1

3. _____ child size

C. No. 2

4. _____ occlusal film size

D. No. 3

5. _____ narrow anterior film size

E. No. 4

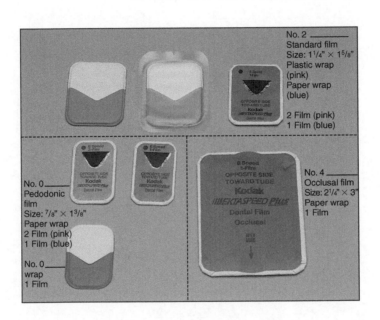

Film Packet

Label the parts of the film packet.

True or false:

_____ Film packets come in double films.

_____ Film packets come in triple films.

_____ Package color and numbering may differ from one manufacturer to another.

_____ Dental film can be stored at high temperatures.

_____ Dental film can be stored in the refrigerator.

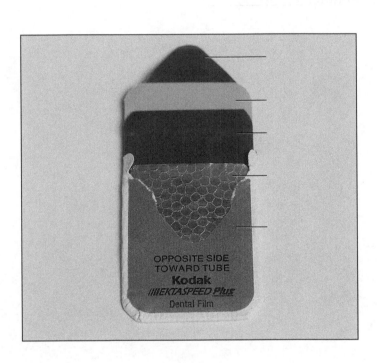

OPPOSITE SIDE
TOWARD TUBE
Kodak
EKTASPEED Plus
Dental Film

Film Holding Devices

Color the RINN bite-wing setup red.

Color the RINN anterior setup blue.

Color the RINN posterior setup yellow.

Color the Snap-A-Ray setup green.

The abbreviation PID stands for _____. Identify some of the film holding devices that are available. _____

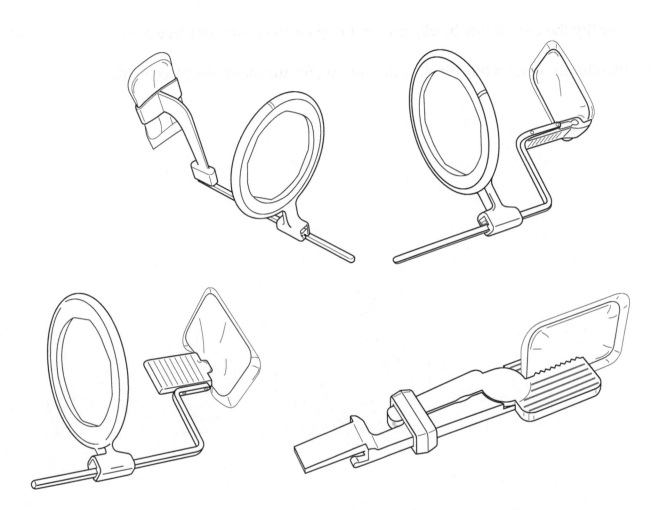

Rinn XCP

Label and color the bite blocks: red for anterior, blue for posterior, and green for bite-wings.

Picking the correct setup:

Identify the correct bite block, arm, and ring for the anterior placement.

Identify the correct bite block, arm, and ring for the posterior placement.

Identify the correct bite block, arm, and ring for the bite-wing placement.

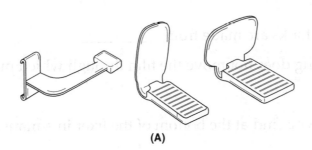

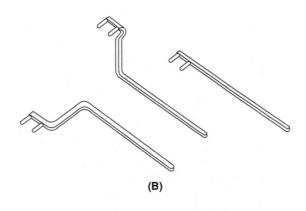

(A)

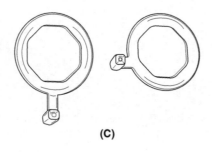

(B)

(C)

Processing Room

Identify and label each of the following in the processing room: automatic processor, silver recovery unit, manual processing tank, thermostatic water control, and safelights.

1. Manual processing tanks are made from _____.

2. Automatic processing does not move the film through which procedure?

   _____

3. What metal would you find at the bottom of the fixer in a manual tank?

   _____

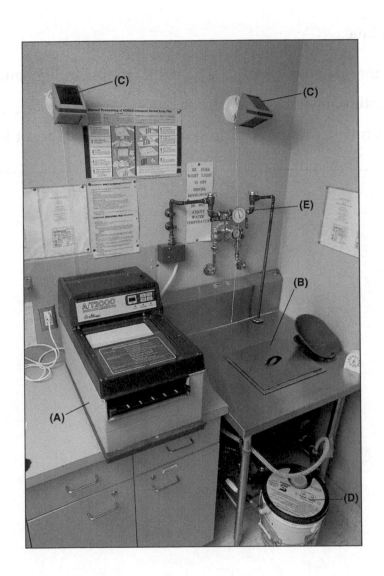

Manual Processing Tank

Label the compartments in the manual processing tank.

Color the developer green.

Color the fixer red.

Color the water blue.

1. Where is the thermometer kept in the dental X-ray processing tank? _____

2. What is the optimum temperature for the processing solution? _____

3. Is the temperature in the automatic processor normally higher or lower than the manual tank? _____

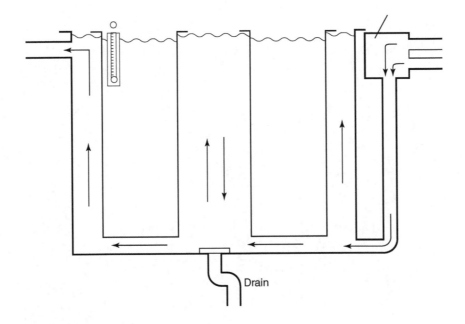

Drain

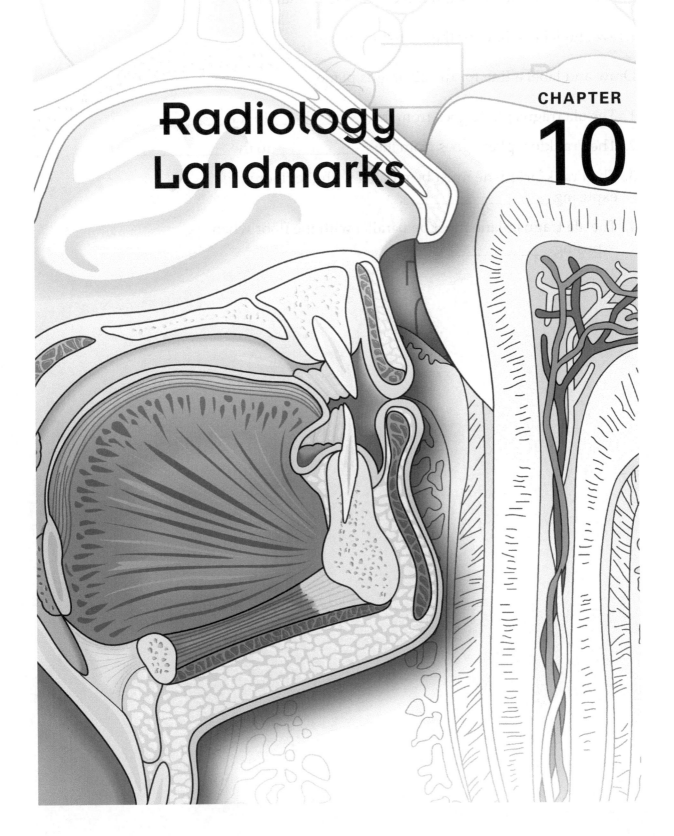

Radiology
Landmarks

Landmark Planes for Exposing Radiographs of the Face

Label a line for the midsagittal plane on the frontal view.

Draw and label a line for the Frankfort plane.

Draw and label a line for the ala tragus plane.

1. The ala tragus plane goes from the _____ to the _____.

2. The Frankfort plane goes from the _____ to the _____.

3. The Frankfort plane must be parallel with the floor when exposing _____.

4. The ala tragus plane must be parallel with the floor when exposing _____.

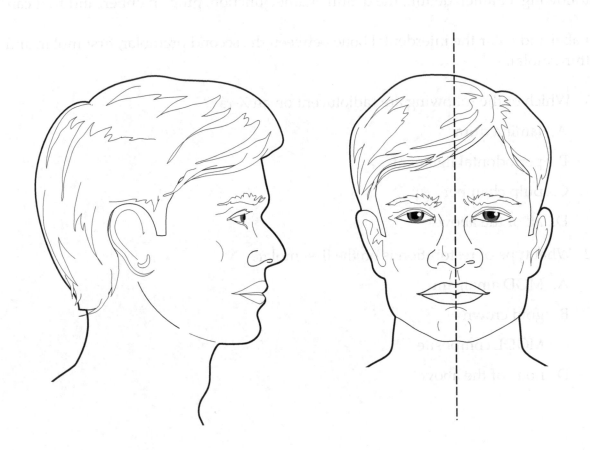

Landmarks for the Tooth and Surrounding Tissues

On the mandibular second premolar, label and color the following: enamel, dentin, pulp, and the pulp chamber.

On the mandibular first molar, label and color the following: cementum, periodontal ligament, lamina dura, root canal, and interradicular bone.

On the mandibular third molar (second molar is missing), label and color the following: enamel, dentin, the dentin enamel junction, pulp chamber, and root canal.

Label and color the interdental bone between the second premolar, first molar, and third molar.

1. Which of the following are radiolucent on an X-ray?

    A. lamina dura

    B. periodontal ligament

    C. pulp chamber

    D. all of the above

2. What type of restoration is on the first molar?

    A. MOD amalgam

    B. gold crown

    C. MODL composite

    D. none of the above

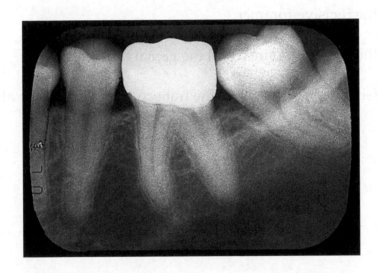

Landmarks for the Surrounding Tissues Continued

Mix and match:

1. lingual foramen   A. raised area of bone surrounding the lingual foramen

2. genial tubercles   B. found on the center of the hard palate

3. trabecular pattern   C. found below the mandibular central incisors

4. incisive foramen   D. spongy appearance of the alveolar bone

Label and outline in color the two maxillary central incisors.

Label and outline in color the two mandibular central incisors.

Label and color the incisive foramen.

Label and color the lingual foramen and the genial tubercles.

Label and color (shade in a light color) the trabecular pattern of the alveolar bone on both X-rays.

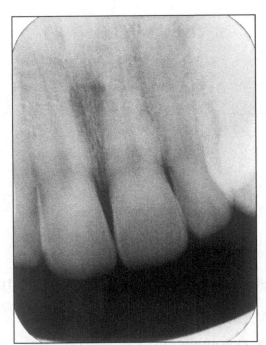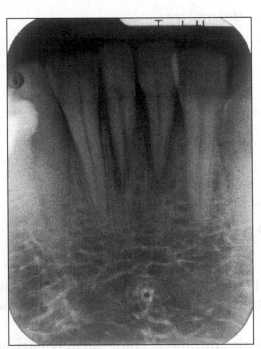

Courtesy of Dr. Rodney Braun and Dr. Chris Chaffin

Landmarks for the Maxillary Arch

1. Which of the following teeth is/are impacted?

    A. right cuspid

    B. left cuspid

    C. right third molar

    D. left third molar

2. The maxillary sinuses are above:

    A. the two central incisors

    B. the molars

    C. the cuspids

    D. the lateral incisors

3. There is overlapping between the _____.

    A. premolars and cuspids

    B. molars

    C. cuspids and laterals

    D. central incisors

Label and outline in color the following: mastoid process, external auditory meatus, and the glenoid fossa on the temporal bone.

Label and outline in color the maxillary sinus, zygomatic process, hard palate, and orbit.

Label and outline in color the nasal fossa, nasal septum, and nasal conchae.

Label and color the incisive foramen and the maxillary tuberosity.

Label the maxillary teeth using the universal system of numbering.

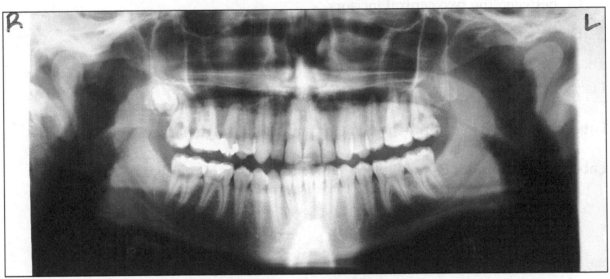

Courtesy of Dr. Rodney Braun and Dr. Chris Chaffin

Landmarks for the Mandibular Arch

1. Which of the following landmarks is part of the temporomandibular joint?

  A. coronoid process

  B. mental foramen

  C. condyle process

  D. retromolar process

2. The mental foramen is located:

  A. behind the last posterior molar

  B. between the first and second molars

  C. between the two central incisors

  D. between the first and second premolars

List, label, and outline in color the parts of the mandible.

Label and outline in color the retromolar pad and the alveolar crest.

Label the mandibular teeth using the universal system of numbering.

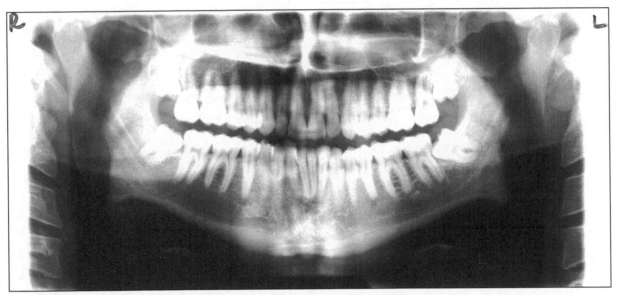

Courtesy of Dr. Rodney Braun and Dr. Chris Chaffin

Miscellaneous

Maslow's Hierarchy of Needs

Color and label each level in Maslow's hierarchy of needs.

Mix and match:

1. _____ bottom layer of Maslow's hierarchy of needs

2. _____ second from the bottom layer of Maslow's hierarchy of needs

3. _____ middle layer of Maslow's hierarchy of needs

4. _____ next to the top layer of Maslow's hierarchy of needs

5. _____ highest layer of Maslow's hierarchy of needs

A. safety needs

B. self-actualization

C. survival or Physiological needs

D. belongingness and Love needs

E. prestige and Esteem needs

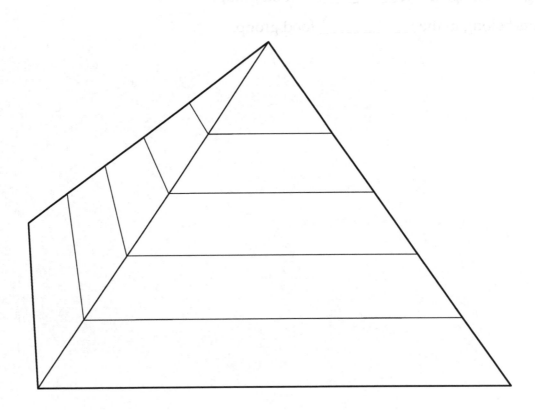

Food Guide Pyramid

Label, color, and identify the servings for each area in the Food Guide Pyramid.

Fill in the blanks:

1. Butter belongs in the _____ food group.

2. Rice and pasta belong in the _____ food group.

3. Bananas and pears belong in the _____ food group.

4. Yogurt belongs in the _____ food group.

5. Nuts belong in the _____ food group.

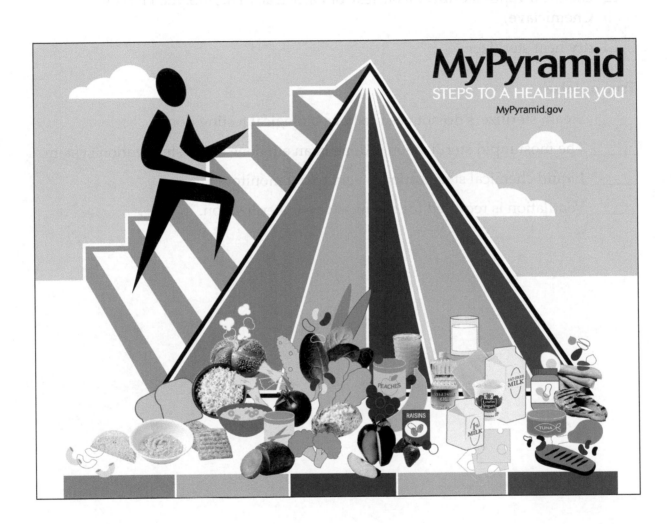

Sterilizers

Match the color of the box to the color of the outside of the box and identify the type of sterilizer and the temperature and time used to process correctly.

☐ steam sterilizer by Statium

☐ Midmark steam sterilizer

☐ chemical vapor sterilizer (courtesy of Barnstead/Thermolyne Harvey Chemiclave)

☐ dry heat sterilizer

True or false:

_____ Steam sterilizers do not need to have biological testing done.

_____ The most rapid sterilization is done in an ethylene oxide sterilization system.

_____ Liquid chemical sterilization is very easily monitored.

_____ Ventilation is required for chemical vapor sterilization.

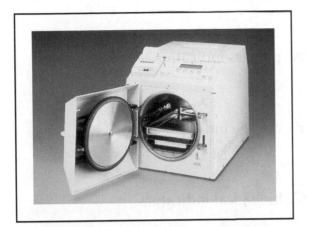

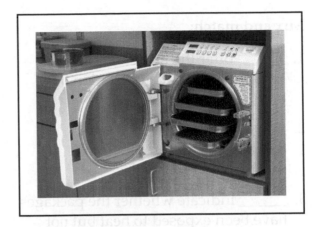

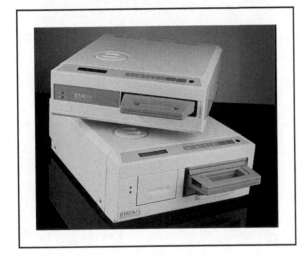

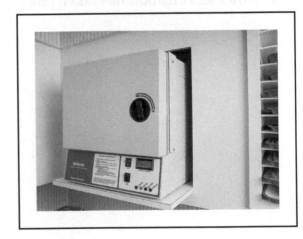

Biological Monitors, Process Indicators, and Dosage Indicators

Label the photos.

Mix and match:

1. _____ offer the most accurate way to assess whether sterilization has occurred

   A. process indicators

2. _____ indicate that correct conditions were present for sterilization to take place

   B. dosage indicators

3. _____ indicate whether the packages have been exposed to heat but not whether sterilization has taken place

   C. biological indicators

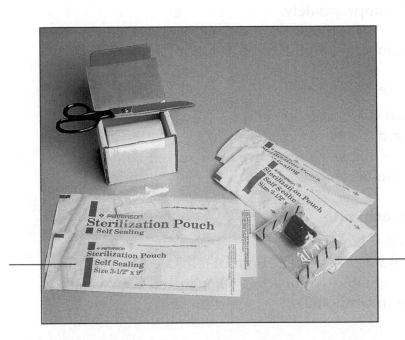

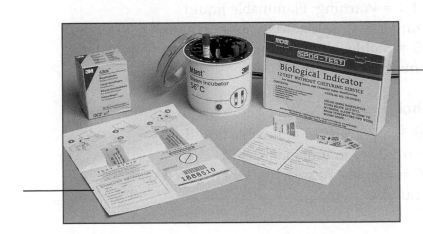

National Fire Protection Association's Color and Number System

Using the four colors of red, yellow, blue, and white that have been developed by the National Fire Protection Association's color and number method, color the labels on the bottles appropriately.

Fill in the numbering on the labels as follows:

Distilled water

Fire Hazard 0 = Noncombustible
Health Hazard 0 = No unusual hazard
Reactivity 0 = Stable: Nonreactive when mixed with water
PPE = (no number noted)

Sodium hypochlorite

Fire Hazard 0 = Noncombustible
Health Hazard 2 = Warning: Harmful if inhaled
Reactivity 0 = Stable: Nonreactive when mixed with water
PPE = (no number noted)

Acetone

Fire Hazard 3 = Warning: Flammable liquid
Health Hazard 1 = Caution: May cause irritation
Reactivity 0 = Stable: Nonreactive when mixed with water
PPE = (no number noted)

Ethyl Alcohol

Fire Hazard 3 = Warning: Flammable liquid
Health Hazard 0 = No unusual hazard
Reactivity 0 = Stable: Nonreactive when mixed with water
PPE = (no number noted)

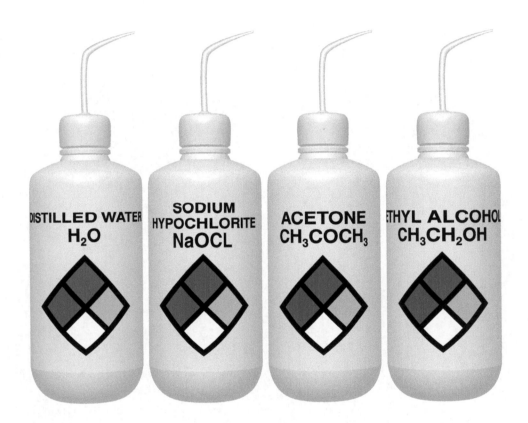

Answer Key

Chapter 1: General Anatomy

Basic Cell Structures

Refer to Figure 6-3 in *Dental Assisting: A Comprehensive Approach 3e*

1. C   2. D   3. A   4. B

Body Planes

Refer to Figure 6-1A in *Dental Assisting: A Comprehensive Approach 3e*

Body Directions

Refer to Figure 6-1B in *Dental Assisting: A Comprehensive Approach 3e*

Body Cavities

Refer to Figure 6-2 in *Dental Assisting: A Comprehensive Approach 3e*

The body cavities are divided into two sections: dorsal and ventral.

The structures in the thoracic cavity include: lungs, heart, and all accessory parts needed for their functioning.

The structures in the abdominal cavity include: digestive tract and supporting organs.

The structures in the pelvic cavity include: urinary bladder, rectum, and reproductive system.

Axial and Appendicular Skeleton

Refer to Figure 6-4 in *Dental Assisting: A Comprehensive Approach 3e*

The axial skeleton includes the skull, spinal column, ribs, and sternum.

The appendicular skeleton includes the upper and lower extremities.

The hands and feet are a part of the appendicular skeleton.

Anatomic Features of Bone

Refer to Figure 6-5 in *Dental Assisting: A Comprehensive Approach 3e*

Spongy bone is also called cancellous bone.

Skeletal Joints

Refer to Figure 6-6 in *Dental Assisting: A Comprehensive Approach 3e*

Another name for joints is articulations.

The temporomandibular joint is a synovial joint.

Types of Muscle Tissue

Refer to Figure 6-7 in *Dental Assisting: A Comprehensive Approach 3e*

1. B   2. C   3. A

Tendons and Ligaments

Refer to Figure 6-8 in *Dental Assisting: A Comprehensive Approach 3e*

Tendons attach muscle to bones.

Ligaments attach or connect bone to bone.

Structure of a Neuron

Refer to Figure 6-9 in *Dental Assisting: A Comprehensive Approach 3e*

Axons conduct impulses away from the nerve cell.

Dendrites conduct impulses toward the nerve cell.

Simple Reflex Arc

Refer to Figure 6-10 in *Dental Assisting: A Comprehensive Approach 3e*

A. Connecting neurons are located in the gray matter.

1. D   2. B   3. A   4. C

Structures of the Endocrine System

Refer to Figure 6-11 in *Dental Assisting: A Comprehensive Approach 3e*

1. C   2. A   3. B   4. D

Systemic and Pulmonary Circulation

Refer to Figure 6-12 in *Dental Assisting: A Comprehensive Approach 3e*

1. B   2. A

Structures of the Heart

Refer to Figure 6-13 in *Dental Assisting: A Comprehensive Approach 3e*

1. B   2. C

Structures of the Digestive System

Refer to Figure 6-14 in *Dental Assisting: A Comprehensive Approach 3e*

1. C   2. D   3. B   4. A

Salivary Glands and Ducts

Refer to Figure 6-14B in *Dental Assisting: A Comprehensive Approach 3e*

The sublingual gland empties directly into the mouth. This gland resembles a tube or hose that lies under the tongue. There are small openings all along this tube for saliva to enter the mouth.

Structures of the Respiratory System

Refer to Figure 6-15 in *Dental Assisting: A Comprehensive Approach 3e*

Bronchial tree is made up of:

- Trachea
- Lung
- Bronchus

Larnyx = voice box

Trachea = windpipe

Epiglottis covers the larynx

Structures of the Bronchi

Refer to Figure 6-15 in *Dental Assisting: A Comprehensive Approach 3e*

Gaseous exchange takes place in the alveoli.

Bronchioles are smaller than the bronchi.

The Lungs

Refer to Figure 6-19 in *Dental Assisting: A Comprehensive Approach 3e*

The lungs lie between the sternum and thoracic vertebrae.

Tonsils

Refer to Figure 6-16 in *Dental Assisting: A Comprehensive Approach 3e*

1. B   2. C   3. A

The Immune System

Refer to Figure 6-17 in *Dental Assisting: A Comprehensive Approach 3e*

1. Spleen

2. Lymph nodes

Chapter 2: Head and Neck Anatomy

Landmarks of the Face

Refer to Figure 7-1 in *Dental Assisting: A Comprehensive Approach 3e*

1. D   2. B   3. A   4. C

Structures of the Oral Cavity–Maxillary View

Refer to Figure 7-2A in *Dental Assisting: A Comprehensive Approach 3e*

1. D. Vestibule fornix

2. Order of tissues starting with the tooth: gingiva, alveolar mucosa, vestibule, and then vestibule fornix

3. Maxillary central incisors

Structures of the Oral Cavity–Mandibular View

Refer to Figure 7-2B in *Dental Assisting: A Comprehensive Approach 3e*

1. A   2. C

Landmarks on the Buccal Mucosa

Refer to Figure 7-3 in *Dental Assisting: A Comprehensive Approach 3e*

1. The linea alba is a raised white tissue found on the buccal mucosa usually reflecting the line of occlusion.

2. "Fordyce's spots" are small glands near the commissures. They are yellowish in color.

Landmarks of the Oral Pharynx Area

Refer to Figure 7-4B in *Dental Assisting: A Comprehensive Approach 3e*

1. B   2. C   3. A

Posterior tonsillar pillars are also called palatopharyngeal arches.

Landmarks of the Palate

Refer to Figure 7-4 in *Dental Assisting: A Comprehensive Approach 3e*

1. Palatine raphe

2. Incisive papilla

3. Palatine rugae

Landmarks on the Dorsal Surface of the Tongue

Refer to Figure 7-5A in *Dental Assisting: A Comprehensive Approach 3e*

Median sulcus

1. B   2. D   3. C   4. A

Landmarks on the Ventral Surface of the Tongue

Refer to Figure 7-5B in *Dental Assisting: A Comprehensive Approach 3e*

C. excess bone formations on the lingual side of the alveolar bone

Basic Taste Buds of the Tongue

Refer to Figure 7-6 in *Dental Assisting: A Comprehensive Approach 3e*

1. Taste buds are stimulated with different chemicals.

2. A

3. The brain

Salivary Glands and Ducts

Refer to Figure 7-7 in *Dental Assisting: A Comprehensive Approach 3e*

1. Sublingual gland

2. Parotid gland

3. Wharton's duct

Lateral Aspect of the Cranium and Face

Refer to Figure 7-8A in *Dental Assisting: A Comprehensive Approach 3e*

Bones of the cranium: Frontal, parietal, occipital, temporal, sphenoid and ethmoid bones.

Bones of the face: nasal, vomer, lacrimal, maxilla, mandible and zygomatic.

1. B. The glenoid fossa is found on the temporal bone

2. A. The vomer

Frontal View of the Bones of the Cranium and Face

Refer to Figure 7-9 in *Dental Assisting: A Comprehensive Approach 3e*

1. C. In the center of the mandible near the border

Landmarks of the Palate

Refer to Figure 7-10 in *Dental Assisting: A Comprehensive Approach 3e*

There are seven foramina on the palate counting the lesser palatine foramina.

Lateral View of the External Surface of the Mandible

Refer to Figure 7-11A in *Dental Assisting: A Comprehensive Approach 3e*

Mix and match:

1. C   2. A   3. D   4. B

There are five foramina in the mandible.

Internal Lingual View of the Mandible

Refer to Figure 7-11B in *Dental Assisting: A Comprehensive Approach 3e*

List the lingual mandibular foramen: Mandibular foramen (2) and lingual foramen (1).

Name the bony raised area surrounding the lingual foramen: genial tubercles.

Another name for the mylohyoid groove is the internal oblique ridge.

Temporomandibular Joint (TMJ)

Refer to Figure 7-12 in *Dental Assisting: A Comprehensive Approach 3e*

B. The condyle is the part of the mandible that makes up the TMJ.

The articular disc (meniscus).

Movement of the Temporomandibular Joint (TMJ)–Hinge Joint

Refer to Figure 7-13A in *Dental Assisting: A Comprehensive Approach 3e*

Meniscus is another name for the articular disc.

The hinge motion occurs when the mandible opens and the condyle and the discs begin rotation anteriorly.

Movement of the Temporomandibur Joint (TMJ)–Gliding Joint

Refer to Figure 7-13B in *Dental Assisting: A Comprehensive Approach 3e*

The gliding motion occurs as the mandible continues to open. The upper and lower cavities of the joint are both involved.

Muscles of Mastication–Lateral View

Refer to Figure 7-14 in *Dental Assisting: A Comprehensive Approach 3e*

Muscles of mastication:

- Masseter
- Temporal
- Internal pterygoid
- External pterygoid

Mix and match:

1. B   2. D   3. A   4. C

Muscles of Facial Expression

Refer to Figure 7-15 in *Dental Assisting: A Comprehensive Approach 3e*

Muscles of facial expression:

- Buccinator muscle
- Mentalis muscle
- Orbicularis oris muscle
- Zygomatic major muscle

The orbicularis oris surrounds the mouth.

D. zygomatic major muscle

B. mentalis muscle

Extrinsic Muscles of the Tongue

Refer to Figure 7-16 in *Dental Assisting: A Comprehensive Approach 3e*

Genioglossus muscle

Hyoglossus muscle

Styloglossus

Palatoglossus

The genioglossus muscle lies across the floor of the mouth.

Muscles of the Floor of the Mouth

Refer to Figure 7-17 in *Dental Assisting: A Comprehensive Approach 3e*

Muscles on the floor of the mouth:

- Geniohyoid
- Mylohyoid
- A. Digastric–anterior belly   B. Digastric–posterior belly
- Styloid

All of these muscles attach to the hyoid bone.

Mix and match:

1. C   2. D   3. A   4. B

The Hyoid Bone

Refer to Figure 7-17B in *Dental Assisting: A Comprehensive Approach 3e*

Fill in answers: mandible vertebrae. or muscles.

Parts of the hyoid bone: greater cornu, lesser cornu, and the body of the hyoid bone.

Muscle groups that are attached to the hyoid bone.

E. muscles of the tongue and muscles on the floor of the mouth.

Muscles of the Soft Palate

Refer to Figure 7-18 in *Dental Assisting: A Comprehensive Approach 3e*

The function of the two muscles of the soft palate is to raise the soft palate during the swallowing process.

C. the palatoglossus muscles are also a part of the muscles of the tongue.

Muscles of the Neck

Refer to Figure 7-19 in *Dental Assisting: A Comprehensive Approach 3e*

Muscles of the neck:

- Platysma
- Sternocleidomastoid
- Trapezius

Mix and match:

1. B   2. A   3. C

The insertion point of each of the muscles of the neck:

- Platysma–inferior border of the mandible
- Sternocleidomastoid–mastoid process anterior part of the occipital bone
- Trapezius–clavicle and shoulders

Nerves of the Maxillary Arch

Refer to Figure 7-20 in *Dental Assisting: A Comprehensive Approach 3e*

1. Posterior superior alveolar nerve

2. Middle superior alveolar nerve

3. Anterior superior alveolar nerve

Mix and match:

1. A   2. C   3. D   4. B

Medial View of the Branches of the Pterygopalatine Nerve

Refer to Figure 7-20B in *Dental Assisting: A Comprehensive Approach 3e*

Branches of the pterygopalatine nerve:

- Greater palatine nerve
- Lesser palatine nerve
- Nasopalatine nerve

Mandibular Nerves

Refer to Figure 7-21 in *Dental Assisting: A Comprehensive Approach 3e*

Three branches of the mandibular nerve:

- Buccal
- Lingual
- Inferior alveolar

Three branches of the inferior alveolar nerve:

- Incisive nerve
- Mental nerve
- Mylohyoid nerve

1. A   2. C   3. A

Arteries of the Face and Oral Cavity

Refer to Figure 7-22 in *Dental Assisting: A Comprehensive Approach 3e*

1. B   2. B

List branches of the external carotid artery:

- Facial artery
- Lingual artery
- Mandibular artery
- Maxillary artery
- Pterygoid artery

List the branches of the mandibular artery:

- Dental arteries
- Incisive arteries
- Inferior alveolar artery
- Mental artery
- Mylohyoid artery

Mix and match:

1. C   2. B   3. D   4. E   5. A

Veins of the Face and Oral Cavity

Refer to Figure 7-23 in *Dental Assisting: A Comprehensive Approach 3e*

1. internal jugular vein

2. superficial veins and deep veins

Superficial veins are: facial, deep facial, retromandibular and lingual.

Deep veins are: maxillary vein and pterygoid plexus of veins.

Chapter 3: Tooth and Tissue Structures

The Three Primary Embryonic Layers

Refer to Figure 8-1 in *Dental Assisting: A Comprehensive Approach 3e*

1. B   2. C   3. A

Embryology

Refer to Figure Table 8-1 in *Dental Assisting: A Comprehensive Approach 3e*

1. Embryonic or germinal stage

2. Zygote phase

3. Embryonic stage

4. Week 4

5. Fetal stage

6. Week 12

Developing Embryo with Primary Layers Identified

Refer to Figure 8-2 in *Dental Assisting: A Comprehensive Approach 3e*

1. Skin, brain, nervous system, hair and nails, enamel of teeth, lining of the oral cavity

2. Epithelial linings, glandular organs, digestive system

3. Bones, muscles, circulatory system, internal organs, reproductive system, lining of the abdominal cavity, dentin, cementum, pulp of the teeth

Facial Processes Shown on an Embryo (Child and Adult)

Refer to Figure 8-3 in *Dental Assisting: A Comprehensive Approach 3e*

Development of the Palate

Refer to Figure 8-4 in *Dental Assisting: A Comprehensive Approach 3e*

1. The primary palate serves to separate the developing oral cavities from the nasal cavitites.

2. The secondary palate contains 6 teeth in each quadrant or 24 teeth total.

Bilaterial Cleft of the Lip (Alveolar Process and Primary Palate)

Refer to Figure 8-10 in *Dental Assisting: A Comprehensive Approach 3e*

1. How many cleft lips occur in 1,000 live births? One

2. Cleft lips are more common in boys or girls? Boys

3. How many cleft palates occur? 1 in every 2,500 births

4. Cleft palates occurring alone are more common in boys or girls? Girls

Life Cycle of the Tooth

Refer to Table 8-2 in *Dental Assisting: A Comprehensive Approach 3e*

Enamel Rods

Refer to Figure 8-13 in *Dental Assisting: A Comprehensive Approach 3e*

1. C   2. B

Tissues of the Tooth

Refer to Figure 8-12 in *Dental Assisting: A Comprehensive Approach 3e*

1. B   2. C   3. D   4. A

Enamel

Refer to Figure 8-14 in *Dental Assisting: A Comprehensive Approach 3e*

1. C   2. D   3. B   4. A

Dentin

Refer to Figure 8-14 in *Dental Assisting: A Comprehensive Approach 3e*

1. C   2. A   3. D   4. B

Pulp

Refer to Figure 8-14 in *Dental Assisting: A Comprehensive Approach 3e*

1. Pulpitis

2. Fibroblasts

3. Intercellular substances

Cementum

Refer to Figure 8-14 in *Dental Assisting: A Comprehensive Approach 3e*

1. T   2. T   3. T   4. F   5. T

Tooth and Surrounding Tissues

Refer to Figure 8-14 in *Dental Assisting: A Comprehensive Approach 3e*

1. Calcified masses of dentin found in pulp tissue, they are quite common

Sharpey's Fibers and Cementum

Refer to Figure 8-15 in *Dental Assisting: A Comprehensive Approach 3e*

Collagen fibers from the periodontal ligament called Sharpey's fibers anchor the tooth to the alveolar bone.

Marginal gingival

Periodontal Ligaments and Alveolar Crests

Refer to Figure 8-16 in *Dental Assisting: A Comprehensive Approach 3e*

1. C   2. A   3. B

Cross-section of Mandibular Molar Tissues of the Tooth Identified

Refer to Figure 8-16 in *Dental Assisting: A Comprehensive Approach 3e*

1. Resist forces that try to pull the tooth outward and resists rotational forces

2. Resist intrusive forces that try to push the tooth inward

3. Function much like the alveolar crest; bigger group but different area

4. Only in multi-rooted teeth, they resist rotational forces and hold the teeth in interproximal contact

5. To resist rotational forces and hold teeth in interproximal contact

6. Resist rotational forces and tilting

Gingival Fiber Groups

Refer to Figure 8-17 in *Dental Assisting: A Comprehensive Approach 3e*

1. In the lamina propria

2. Aid in attaching the gingiva to the alveolar bone

3. Circle and tighten the gingival margin around the neck of the tooth

4. Support fibers that anchor the tooth to the bone

5. Support fibers that anchor the tooth to the bone

Periodontium

Refer to Figure 8-18 in *Dental Assisting: A Comprehensive Approach 3e*

Interdental gingiva or interdental papilla.

Interdental gingiva, gingival sulcus, epithelial attachment.

Marginal gingiva.

Alveolar Mucosa

Refer to Figure 8-19 in *Dental Assisting: A Comprehensive Approach 3e*

1. Attached gingiva

2. Interdental gingiva/interdental papilla

3. Epithelial attachments

4. Mucogingival junction, alveolar mucosa

5. Gingival groove

6. Gingival sulcus

Chapter 4: Tooth Anatomy

Adult Dentition

Refer to Figure 9-2 and 9-4 in *Dental Assisting: A Comprehensive Approach 3e*

Deciduous Dentition

Refer to Figure 9-4 in *Dental Assisting: A Comprehensive Approach 3e*

1. C   2. I   3. D   4. A   5. E

6. B   7. J   8. F   9. H   10. G

Primary Dentition

Refer to Figure 9-2 in *Dental Assisting: A Comprehensive Approach 3e*

Permanent Dentition

Refer to Figure 9-2 in *Dental Assisting: A Comprehensive Approach 3e*

Primary Teeth

Refer to Figure 9-4 in *Dental Assisting: A Comprehensive Approach 3e*

Permanent Dentition

Refer to Figure 9-3 in *Dental Assisting: A Comprehensive Approach 3e*

Permanent Dentition

Refer to Figure 9-8 in *Dental Assisting: A Comprehensive Approach 3e*

Permanent Dentition

Refer to Figure 9-8 in *Dental Assisting: A Comprehensive Approach 3e*

Permanent Dentition

Refer to Figure 9-8 in *Dental Assisting: A Comprehensive Approach 3e*

1. E   2. A   3. F   4. B

5. C   6. II   7. G   8. D

Anatomical Structures

Refer to Figure 9-28 in *Dental Assisting: A Comprehensive Approach 3e*

Anatomical Landmarks

Refer to Figure 9-17, 9-21, 9-23, 9-25 in *Dental Assisting: A Comprehensive Approach 3e*

Anatomical Landmarks

Refer to Figure 9-12 in *Dental Assisting: A Comprehensive Approach 3e*

Match the structure to the definition. Label and color the structure on the illustration.

1. B   2. A   3. F   4. E   5. C   6. D

Maxillary Central Incisors

Refer to Figure 9-32 in *Dental Assisting: A Comprehensive Approach 3e*

Has imbrication lines

First tooth from the midline

Play an important part in appearance

Longest crown in maxillary arch

Play an important part in speech

Used for cutting food

Mesial surface is longer than the distal surface

When erupted it has mamelons

Root inclines to the distal slightly

Labial surface convex

Has a cingulum

Root is 1½ the size of the crown

One root

Blunt apex

Mesial angle acute

Maxillary Lateral Incisors

Refer to Figure 9-34 in *Dental Assisting: A Comprehensive Approach 3e*

1. C   2. B   3. A

Maxillary Canine

Refer to Figure 9-35 in *Dental Assisting: A Comprehensive Approach 3e*

1. Cornerstone of the mouth

2. Tear the food

3. Longest

Maxillary First Bicuspid (Premolar)

Refer to Figure 9-36 in *Dental Assisting: A Comprehensive Approach 3e*

Cusps come together on the occlusal surface in a central groove

It is bifurcated

Posterior tooth

Function is to pulverize food

Removed for ortho sometimes

Buccal cusp is longer than the lingual

Maxillary Second Bicuspid (Premolar)

Refer to Figure 9-37 in *Dental Assisting: A Comprehensive Approach 3e*

1. False

2. False

3. False

4. True

5. False

Maxillary First Molar

Refer to Figure 9-38 in *Dental Assisting: A Comprehensive Approach 3e*

1. _____ single root __✓__ bifurcated _____ trifurcated

2. __✓__ erupts 6 yrs of age _____ erupts 12 years of age _____ erupts 18 years of age

3. _____ tear _____ pulverize __✓__ chew

4. _____ 3 cusps _____ 4 cusps __✓__ 5 cusps

5. __✓__ cusp of Carabelli _____ no cusp of Carabelli

6. _____ roots together __✓__ roots spread apart

Maxillary Second Molar

Refer to Figure 9-39 in *Dental Assisting: A Comprehensive Approach 3e*

1. 4

2. 3

3. Smaller

4. 12

5. Millstone

Maxillary Third Molar

Refer to Figure 9-40 in *Dental Assisting: A Comprehensive Approach 3e*

1. 17–21 years

2. Wisdom, because it was thought that by the time these teeth erupted into the oral cavity a person would have obtained maturity or wisdom

3. No

4. Supplemental

5. Removed

Mandibular Central Incisors

Refer to Figure 9-41 in *Dental Assisting: A Comprehensive Approach 3e*

1. Mandibular

2. Mandibular

3. Mandibular

4. Both

5. Both

Mandibular Lateral Incisors

Refer to Figure 9-42 in *Dental Assisting: A Comprehensive Approach 3e*

1. True

2. True

3. False

4. False

Mandibular Cuspids

Refer to Figure 9-43 in *Dental Assisting: A Comprehensive Approach 3e*

Third tooth from the midline

Not as well-developed as the maxillary canine

Longest tooth in the mandibular arch

One canal in the root

Cornerstone for the mandibular arch

Mandibular First Bicuspids (Premolars)

Refer to Figure 9-44 in *Dental Assisting: A Comprehensive Approach 3e*

Mandibular Second Bicuspids (Premolars)

Refer to Figure 9-45 in *Dental Assisting: A Comprehensive Approach 3e*

1. B   2. C   3. A   4. D

Mandibular First Molar

Refer to Figure 9-46 in *Dental Assisting: A Comprehensive Approach 3e*

Label and color the mandibular first molars.

Color a red box around each item that refers to mandibular first molar: bifurcated, no cusps of Carabelli.

Color a blue box around each item that refers to maxillary first molar: trifurcated, cusp of Carabelli.

Color a green box around each item that refers to both maxillary and mandibular first molars: erupts 6 years of age, chew, 5 cusps, roots spread apart, buccal groove, lingual groove.

Mandibular Second Molar

Refer to Figure 9-47 in *Dental Assisting: A Comprehensive Approach 3e*

Mix and match:

mandibular first molar ——————————— bifurcated and spread apart the most
mandibular first molar —————————— bifurcated and roots closer together
mandibular second molar —————————— may have many roots
mandibular second molar —————————— 6 year molar
mandibular third molar —————————— 12 year molar
mandibular third molar ——————————— wisdom tooth

Mandibular Third Molar

Refer to Figure 9-48 in *Dental Assisting: A Comprehensive Approach 3e*

1. Wisdom teeth

2. Distal

3. Horizontal

Mixed Dentition of a Seven- or Eight-Year-Old

Refer to Figure 9-5 in *Dental Assisting: A Comprehensive Approach 3e*

Contact and Embrasure

Refer to Figure 9-11 in *Dental Assisting: A Comprehensive Approach 3e*

Deciduous Maxillary Teeth

Refer to Figure 9-1 in *Dental Assisting: A Comprehensive Approach 3e*

Deciduous Mandibular Teeth

Refer to Figure 9-1 in *Dental Assisting: A Comprehensive Approach 3e*

1. E   2. B   3. C   4. A   5. D

Identification of Teeth

Refer to Figure 9-1 in *Dental Assisting: A Comprehensive Approach 3e*

Eruption Dates for Primary Teeth

1. Emerges into the oral cavity

2. Maxillary and mandibular first molar

3. Maxillary and mandibular central incisor

4. Maxillary second molar

5. Maxillary lateral incisor

6. Maxillary and mandibular Canine

Exfoliation Dates for Primary Teeth

1. Shed from the oral cavity

2. Maxillary and mandibular central incisor

3. Maxillary canine/maxillary and mandibular second molar

4. Maxillary and mandibular first molar

5. Maxillary and mandibular lateral incisor

Chapter 5: Dental Charting

Universal Numbering System

Refer to Figure 14-1 and 14-2 in *Dental Assisting: A Comprehensive Approach 3e*

__#3__ maxillary right first molar

__#20__ mandibular left second bicuspid (premolar)

___#10___ maxillary left lateral incisor

___#6___ maxillary right cuspid

___#32___ mandibular right third molar

International Standards of Organization Numbering System

Refer to Figure 14-3 and 14-4 in *Dental Assisting: A Comprehensive Approach 3e*

___C.___ maxillary right third molar   A. tooth #25

___B.___ mandibular left central incisor   B. tooth #31

___D.___ mandibular right central incisor   C. tooth #18

___A.___ maxillary left second bicuspid (premolar)   D. tooth #41

Palmer Numbering System

Refer to Figure 14-5 and 14-6 in *Dental Assisting: A Comprehensive Approach 3e*

___3|___ maxillary right cuspid

___6|___ mandibular right first molar

___|2___ maxillary left lateral incisor

___|7___ maxillary left second molar

___|4___ mandibular left first bicuspid (premolar)

Charting Example #1

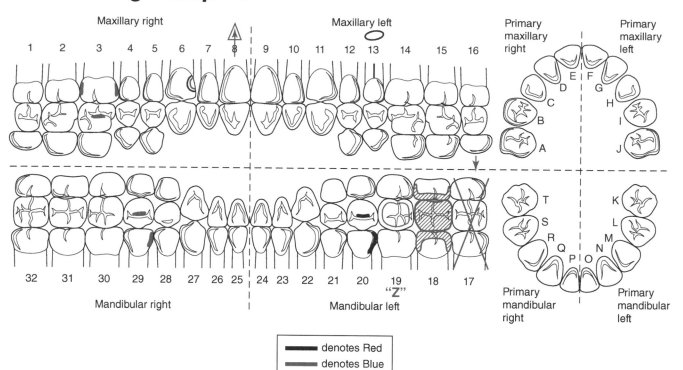

Maxillary right | Maxillary left

Primary maxillary right | Primary maxillary left

1 2 3 4 5 6 7 8 | 9 10 11 12 13 14 15 16

E F
D G
C H
B I
A J

Mandibular right | Mandibular left

32 31 30 29 28 27 26 25 | 24 23 22 21 20 19 18 17

"Z"

Primary mandibular right | Primary mandibular left

T K
S L
R M
Q N
P O

━━━ denotes Red
━━━ denotes Blue

Charting Example #2

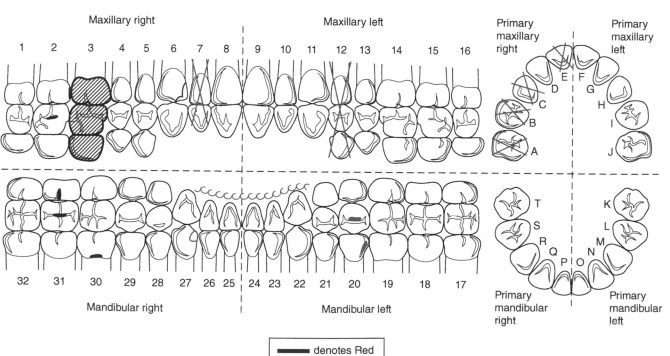

Maxillary right | Maxillary left

Primary maxillary right | Primary maxillary left

1 2 3 4 5 6 7 8 | 9 10 11 12 13 14 15 16

E F
D G
C H
B I
A J

Mandibular right | Mandibular left

32 31 30 29 28 27 26 25 | 24 23 22 21 20 19 18 17

Primary mandibular right | Primary mandibular left

T K
S L
R M
Q N
P O

━━━ denotes Red
━━━ denotes Blue

Charting Example #3

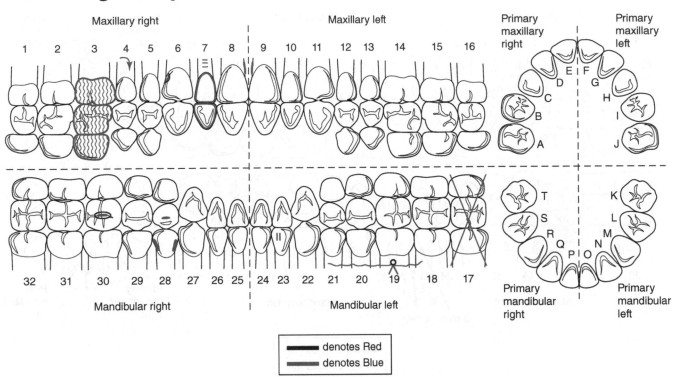

Charting Example #4

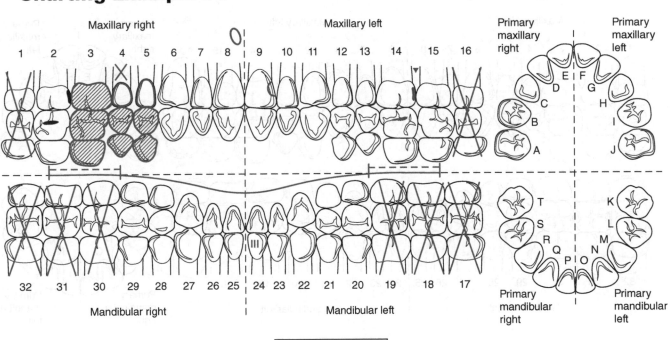

Charting Example #5

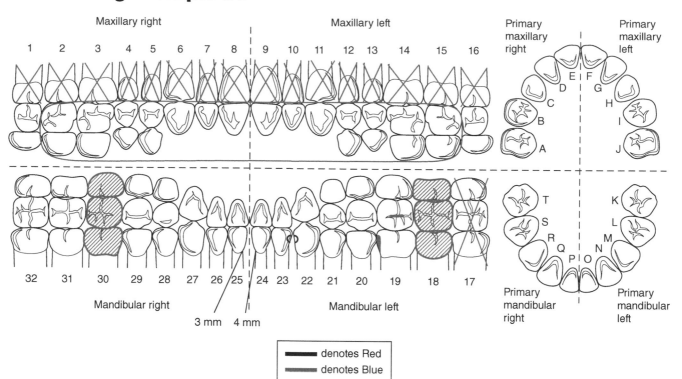

| | | denotes Red |
| | | denotes Blue |

Charting Example #6

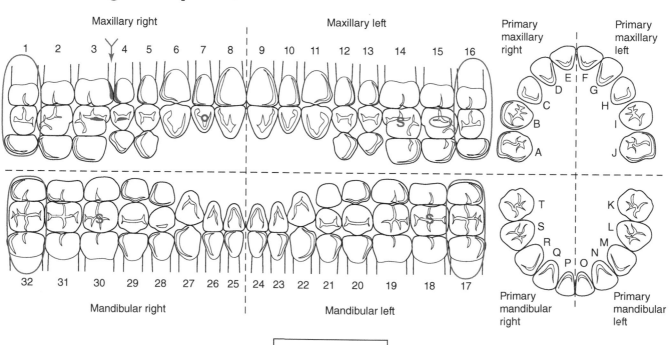

| | | denotes Red |
| | | denotes Blue |

Charting Example #7

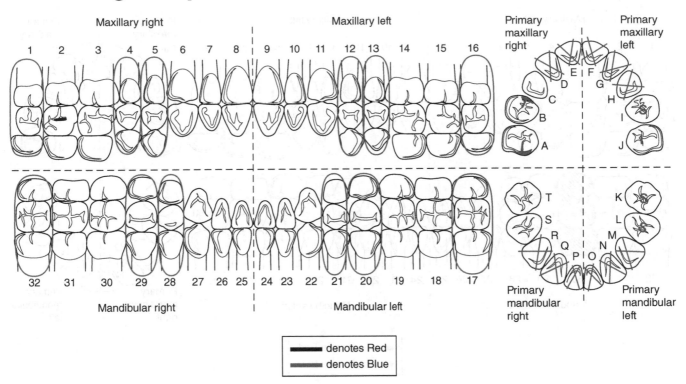

Maxillary right — Maxillary left

1 2 3 4 5 6 7 8 | 9 10 11 12 13 14 15 16

32 31 30 29 28 27 26 25 | 24 23 22 21 20 19 18 17

Mandibular right — Mandibular left

Primary maxillary right — Primary maxillary left

E F
D G
C H
B I
A J

T K
S L
R M
Q N
P O

Primary mandibular right — Primary mandibular left

▬▬▬ denotes Red
▬▬▬ denotes Blue

Charting Example #8

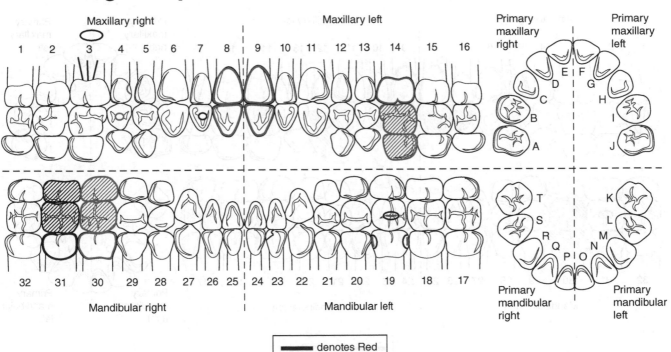

Maxillary right — Maxillary left

1 2 3 4 5 6 7 8 | 9 10 11 12 13 14 15 16

32 31 30 29 28 27 26 25 | 24 23 22 21 20 19 18 17

Mandibular right — Mandibular left

Primary maxillary right — Primary maxillary left

E F
D G
C H
B I
A J

T K
S L
R M
Q N
P O

Primary mandibular right — Primary mandibular left

▬▬▬ denotes Red
▬▬▬ denotes Blue

Charting Example #9

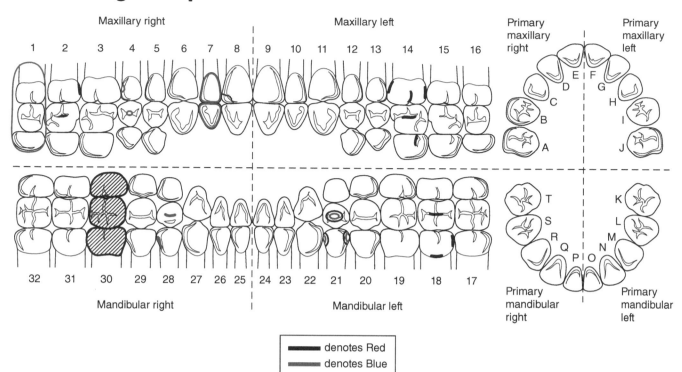

Maxillary right   Maxillary left   Primary maxillary right   Primary maxillary left

1 2 3 4 5 6 7 8 | 9 10 11 12 13 14 15 16

E F
D G
C H
B I
A J

32 31 30 29 28 27 26 25 | 24 23 22 21 20 19 18 17

Mandibular right   Mandibular left   Primary mandibular right   Primary mandibular left

T K
S L
R M
Q N
P O

━━━ denotes Red
━━━ denotes Blue

Charting Example #10

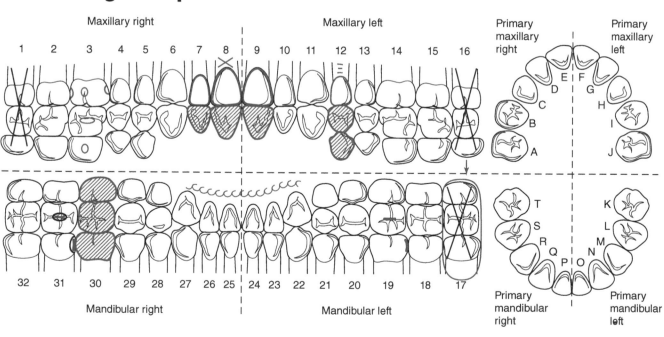

Maxillary right   Maxillary left   Primary maxillary right   Primary maxillary left

1 2 3 4 5 6 7 8 | 9 10 11 12 13 14 15 16

E F
D G
C H
B I
A J

32 31 30 29 28 27 26 25 | 24 23 22 21 20 19 18 17

Mandibular right   Mandibular left   Primary mandibular right   Primary mandibular left

T K
S L
R M
Q N
P O

━━━ denotes Red
━━━ denotes Blue

Chapter 6: Introduction to the Dental Office and Basic Chairside Assisting

Small Dental Office Blueprint

Refer to Figure 17-1 in *Dental Assisting: A Comprehensive Approach 3e*

1. There are three treatment rooms.

Type of equipment found in the treatment rooms: curing light, amalgamator, x-ray view box, communication system, and computer.

Mix and match:

1. D   2. E   3. B   4. C   5. A

Sterilization Area

Refer to Figure 17-5 in *Dental Assisting: A Comprehensive Approach 3e*

Items found in sterilizing area:

- Sink
- Countertop space
- Ultrasonic unit
- Sterilizing units
- Storage
- Handpiece cleaning unit
- Hazardous waste container
- Sharps container

Laboratory Area

Refer to Figure 17-6 in *Dental Assisting: A Comprehensive Approach 3e*

1. Dental lathe or a laboratory handpiece

2. Vibrator and model trimmer

3. Four other items found in the dental lab include: rubber bowls and spatulas, laboratory handpiece, plaster/stone storage bins, and heat source and exhaust fan

Dental Treatment Room

Refer to Figure 17-9 in *Dental Assisting: A Comprehensive Approach 3e*

Procedure trays are stored behind the patient chair, above the cabinet countertop.

Operator's Mobile Cart

Refer to Figure 17-16 in *Dental Assisting: A Comprehensive Approach 3e*

Mix and match:

1. C   2. A   3. D   4. B

Air-water Syringe

Refer to Figure 17-17 in *Dental Assisting: A Comprehensive Approach 3e*

The functions of the air-water syringe include providing air, providing water, or providing a combination of air and water spray. This helps to keep the oral cavity clean and dry during procedures.

1. Only the air-water syringe tips can be sterilized

2. Yes, the tips are removable

3. Yes, disposible tips are available

4. The air-water syringe is flushed with water between patients and at the beginning of the day

Activity Zones

Refer to Figure 17-28 in *Dental Assisting: A Comprehensive Approach 3e*

1. D. all of the above

2. D. —static zone

3. A. —right-handed operator

Chapter 7: Basic Chairside Instruments and Tray Systems

Parts of an Instrument and Different Shanks

Refer to Figure 19-1 and 19-4 in *Dental Assisting: A Comprehensive Approach 3e*

1. straight

2. curved

3. monangle

4. binangle

5. triple angle

1. Posterior areas of the mouth

2. Anterior areas of the mouth

Instruments with Black's Three-Number Formula

Refer to Figure 19-6 in *Dental Assisting: A Comprehensive Approach 3e*

1. First number is the width of the blade in tenths of a millimeter

2. Second number is the length of the blade in millimeters

3. Third number is the angle of the blade to the long axis of the handle, in degrees centigrade

Three number instruments: chisels, hatchets, and hoes.

Instruments with Black's Four-Number Formula

Refer to Figure 19-7 in *Dental Assisting: A Comprehensive Approach 3e*

1. First number is the width of the blade in tenths of a millimeter

2. Second number is the degree of the angle from the cutting edge of the blade to the handle of the instrument

3. Third number is the length of the blade in millimeters

4. Fourth number is the angle of the blade to the long axis of the handle, in degrees Centigrade

Four number instruments: gingival margin trimmers and angle formers.

Chisels, Hatchets, and Hoes

Refer to Figure 19-9, 19-11, and 19-10 in *Dental Assisting: A Comprehensive Approach 3e*

Chisels: straight, Wedelstaedt, and binangle.

1. Cutting instruments

2. Hatchets

3. Wedelstaedt

4. A. beveled edge

Gingival Margin Trimmers and Angle Formers

Refer to Figure 19-13 and 19-12 in *Dental Assisting: A Comprehensive Approach 3e*

1. C. four-number instrument in Black's formula

2. The second number

3. Distal

Excavators

Refer to Figure 19-14 in *Dental Assisting: A Comprehensive Approach 3e*

1. Spoon excavators

2. Blade and spoon excavators

3. B. remove carious debris from the tooth

Explorers, Periodontal Probe, and Cotton Pliers

Refer to Figure 19-16, 19-17, and 19-18 in *Dental Assisting: A Comprehensive Approach 3e*

1. Locking pliers

2. Expro

Cement Spatulas and Burnishers

Refer to Figure 19-23 and 19-26 in *Dental Assisting: A Comprehensive Approach 3e*

Burnishers are used to:

D. smooth margins on restorations and smooth metal matrix bands

Condensors, Carvers, and Plastic Filling Instruments

Refer to Figure 19-19, 19-21, and 19-22 in *Dental Assisting: A Comprehensive Approach 3e*

Mix and match:

1. D   2. A   3. B   4. C

Parts of a Bur and Shanks

Refer to Figure 19-29 in *Dental Assisting: A Comprehensive Approach 3e*

Three types of shanks:

Straight

Latch-type

Friction grip

Friction grip shank is used with a high speed handpiece.

Straight shank is used with a slow speed handpiece without an attachment.

Cutting Bur Shapes and Number Ranges

Refer to Figure 19-30 in *Dental Assisting: A Comprehensive Approach 3e*

List the cutting burs:

Round	Plain tapered fissure
Inverted cone	Plain fissure straight
Crosscut fissure straight	Crosscut fissure tapered
End cutting	Wheel
Pear	

Mix and match:

1. C   2. E   3. D   4. A   5. B

Mix and match:

1. B   2. A   3. D   4. C

Diamond Burs, Finishing Burs, Surgical Burs, and Laboratory Burs

Refer to Figure 19-31, 19-32, 19-33, and 19-34 in *Dental Assisting: A Comprehensive Approach 3e*

1. B   2. C

3. A. the diamond burs
   D. the laboratory burs

High- and Low-speed Handpieces and Attachments

Refer to Figure 19-42 and 19-43 in *Dental Assisting: A Comprehensive Approach 3e*

1. High-speed handpiece

2. Prophy angle

3. Chuck

4. Rheostat

5. Straight

Double Color-coding

Procedure

Treatment room

Operator—dentist/hygienist

Different set of the same instruments for the same procedure

Triple Color-coding

Triple color-coding is used In larger dental offices, where one or more dentists and several hygienists work.

Triple color-coding can designate the procedure, treatment room/operator, and individual set of instruments.

Color-coding for Procedure Sequence

Benefits for procedure color coding:

Indicating the sequence of a procedure allows the procedure to move faster

Makes setting up trays easier for new auxillary, interns, and temporary assistants

Chapter 8: Anesthesia and Sedation

Types of Anesthetic Injections

Refer to Figure Figures 20-3, 20-4, and 20-5 in *Dental Assisting: A Comprehensive Approach 3e*

Local infiltration

Field block anesthesia

Nerve block anesthesia

The nerve block anesthesia is the injection that is close to a main nerve trunk.

The local infiltration places anesthetic solution into the tissues near the small terminal nerve branches.

Maxillary Arch Injections and Site Locations

Refer to Figure 20-6 in *Dental Assisting: A Comprehensive Approach 3e*

1. E   2. A   3. D   4. B   5. F   6. C

Mandibular Arch Injections and Site Locations

Refer to Figure 20-7 in *Dental Assisting: A Comprehensive Approach 3e*

1. Buccal nerve block

2. Incisive nerve block

3. Inferior alveolar nerve block

4. Lingual nerve block

5. Mental nerve block

1. Inferior alveolar nerve block

2. Incisive nerve block and mental nerve block

3. Buccal, lingual, and inferior alveolar nerve block

Aspirating Syringe

Refer to Figure 20-8 in *Dental Assisting: A Comprehensive Approach 3e*

Plunger is another name for a piston rod.

A. False statement

Needle Parts

Refer to Figure 20-9 in *Dental Assisting: A Comprehensive Approach 3e*

1. B. a long needle is used for a block injection

2. A. toward the tissues/bone

3. C. either metal or plastic

Parts of an Anesthetic Cartridge

Refer to Figure 20-11A in *Dental Assisting: A Comprehensive Approach 3e*

- Aluminum cap
- Glass cylinder
- Neck
- Rubber diaphragm
- Rubber stopper

Four things to look for before using an anesthetic syringe:

- Expired shelf-life dates
- Large bubbles
- Extruded plungers
- Corrosion or rust around the aluminum cap

or cracks around the neck region and the rubber stopper area.

The diaphragm is located on the syringe end of the cartridge.

Information on the Anesthetic Cartridge

Refer to Figure 20-11B in *Dental Assisting: A Comprehensive Approach 3e*

Information found on the glass cylinder of an anesthetic syringe:

brand name, solution concentration, volume of anesthetic, vasoconstrictor ratio (if solution contains a vasoconstrictor), lot number and expiration date.

Mix and match:

1. C   2. A   3. D   4. B

Equipment and Supplies Needed to Prepare an Anesthetic Syringe

Refer to Figure 20-13 in *Dental Assisting: A Comprehensive Approach 3e*

Chapter 9: Dental X-Ray Film and Holding Devices

Electromagnetic Energy Spectrum and Applications

Refer to Figure 21-4 in *Dental Assisting: A Comprehensive Approach 3e*

Primary, Secondary and Leakage Radiation

Refer to Figure 21-5 in *Dental Assisting: A Comprehensive Approach 3e*

Mix and match:

1. C. red primary radiation

2. D. blue secondary radiation

3. A. yellow leakage radiation

4. B. green scatter radiation

Parts of Dental Arm Assembly

Refer to Figure 21-8 in *Dental Assisting: A Comprehensive Approach 3e*

1. Extension arm assembly

2. Tube head

3. Position indicator device

4. Control panel

Tube Head, PID, Vertical Indicator Scale

Refer to Figure 21-8B in *Dental Assisting: A Comprehensive Approach 3e*

E	Y	A	U	R	S	X	T	B
S	T	X	Y	A	B	R	U	E
U	R	B	T	E	X	A	Y	S
X	E	R	S	U	T	B	A	Y
A	U	T	B	Y	E	S	X	R
Y	B	S	R	X	A	U	E	T
B	A	Y	X	T	R	E	S	U
T	S	E	A	B	U	Y	R	X
R	X	U	E	S	Y	T	B	A

Tube Head and X-Ray Tube

Refer to Figure 21-12 in *Dental Assisting: A Comprehensive Approach 3e*

1. Cathode

2. Anode

3. Cathode

4. Anode

5. Anode

X-ray Tube

1. Diaphragm

2. Central beam

3. Focal spot

Composition of Dental X-ray Film

Refer to Figure 21-13 in *Dental Assisting: A Comprehensive Approach 3e*

1. 0.2 mm

2. Bluish

3. Cellulose acetate

Sizes of Dental X-ray Film

Refer to Figure 21-14 in *Dental Assisting: A Comprehensive Approach 3e*

Label the film sizes and color on the illustration

Mix and match:

adult size   C. No. 2

long bite-wing film size   D. No. 3

child size   A. No. 0

occlusal film size   E. No. 4

narrow anterior film size   B. No. 1

Film Packet

Refer to Figure 21-5 in *Dental Assisting: A Comprehensive Approach 3e*

Label the parts of the film packet: Outer package and black paper, dental film, black paper, lead foil backing, outer package.

True or false:

T   Film packets come in double films.

F   Film packets come in triple films.

T   Package color and numbering may differ from one manufacturer to another.

F   Dental film can be stored at high temperatures.

T   Dental film can be stored in the refrigerator.

Film Holding Devices

Refer to Figure 22-10 in *Dental Assisting: A Comprehensive Approach 3e*

The abbreviation PID stands for position indicator device.

Identify some of the film holding devices that are available: RINN, Snap-a-ray.

Rinn XCP

Refer to Figure 22-11 in *Dental Assisting: A Comprehensive Approach 3e*

Processing Room

Refer to Figure 22-34 in *Dental Assisting: A Comprehensive Approach 3e*

1. Stainless steel

2. Additional water after development

3. Silver

Manual Processing Tank

Refer to Figure 22-33B in *Dental Assisting: A Comprehensive Approach 3e*

1. Developer

2. 68 degrees–70 degrees Farenheit

3. Higher

Chapter 10: Radiology Landmarks

Landmark Planes for Exposing Radiographs of the Face

Refer to Figure 23-10 in *Dental Assisting: A Comprehensive Approach 3e*

1. Ala of the nose (flared side of nostril) to tragus of the ear (center of the ear)

2. Bridge of the nose just below the eye to the middle of the ear (tragus)

3. Mandibular arch

4. Maxillary arch

Landmarks for the Tooth and Surrounding Tissues

Refer to Figure 23-22 in *Dental Assisting: A Comprehensive Approach 3e*

1. D   2. B

Landmarks for the Surrounding Tissues

Refer to Figure 23-24B and 23-23B in *Dental Assisting: A Comprehensive Approach 3e*

Mix and match:

1. C   2. A   3. D   4. B

Landmarks for the Maxillary Arch

Refer to Figure 23-24 in *Dental Assisting: A Comprehensive Approach 3e*

1. C   2. B   3. A

Landmarks for the Mandibular Arch

Refer to Figure 10-5 in *Dental Assisting: A Comprehensive Approach 3e*

1. C   2. D

Parts of the mandible:

- Condyle process
- Coronoid process
- Border of the mandible
- Symphysis
- Medial sigmoid notch
- Ramus
- Mental foramen
- Mandibular canal
- Mandibular foramen
- External oblique ridge
- Angle of the mandible

Chapter 11: Miscellaneous

Maslow's Hierarchy of Needs

Refer to Figure 2-6 in *Dental Assisting: A Comprehensive Approach 3e*

1. C   2. A   3. D   4. E   5. B

Food Guide Pyramid

Refer to Figure 5-2 in *Dental Assisting: A Comprehensive Approach 3e*

1. Fats, oils, and sweets

2. Bread, cereal, rice, and pasta

3. Fruit

4. Milk, yogurt, and cheese

5. Meat, poultry, fish, dry beans, eggs, and nuts

Sterilizers

Refer to Figure 11-17, 11-18, 11-19, and 11-20 in *Dental Assisting: A Comprehensive Approach 3e*

True or false:

F   Steam sterilizers do not need to have biological testing done.

F   The most rapid sterilization is done in an ethylene oxide sterilization system.

F   Liquid chemical sterilization is very easily monitored.

T   Ventilation is required for chemical vapor sterilization.

Biological Monitors, Process Indicators, and Dosage Indicators

Refer to Figure 11-22 in *Dental Assisting: A Comprehensive Approach 3e*

1. C   2. B   3. A

National Fire Protection Association's Color and Number System

Refer to Figure 12-12 in *Dental Assisting: A Comprehensive Approach 3e*